Dilemmas in UK Health Care

Edited by Carol Komaromy

Published by Open University Press

Produced by The Open University

Health and Disease Series, Book 7

OPEN UNIVERSITY PRESS

Buckingham • Philadelphia

The Open University

The U205 *Health and Disease* Course Team

The following members of the Open University teaching staff have collaborated with the authors in writing this book, or have commented extensively on it during its production. We accept collective responsibility for its overall academic and teaching content.

Basiro Davey (Course Team Chair, Senior Lecturer in Health Studies, Department of Biological Sciences)

Linda Jones (Senior Lecturer, School of Health and Social Welfare)

Carol Komaromy (Lecturer in Health Studies, School of Health and Social Welfare)

Moyra Sidell (Senior Lecturer, School of Health and Social Welfare)

The following people have contributed to the development of particular parts or aspects of this book.

Gerry Bearman (editor)

Celia Davies (critical reader) Professor of Health Care, School of Health and Social Welfare, The Open University

Sheila Dunleavy (editor)

Phil Gauron (BBC producer)

Rebecca Graham (editor)

Tanya Hames (secretary)

Celia Hart (picture researcher)

Pam Higgins (designer)

Mike Levers (photographer)

Jean Macqueen (indexer)

Jennifer Nockles (designer)

Dick Sharp (editor)

Sue Spurr (course manager)

John Taylor (graphic artist)

Judy Thomas (librarian)

Geoff Wheeler (BBC producer)

Joy Wilson (course manager)

Authors

The following people have acted as principal authors for the chapters listed below.

Chapters 1 and 7

Carol Komaromy, Lecturer in Health Studies, School of Health and Social Welfare, The Open University.

Chapter 2

Alan Williams, Professor of Economics, Centre for Health Economics, University of York.

Chapter 3

David Cox, Professor and Associate Dean (Academic) Health and Community Care, University of Central England.

Chapter 4

Bob Hudson, Principal Research Fellow, Community Care Division, Nuffield Institute, University of Leeds.

Chapter 5

Carole Thornley, Senior Lecturer in Industrial Relations, Department of Human Resource Management and Industrial Relations, University of Keele.

Chapter 6

David Foxcroft, Professor of Health Care Practice, Oxford Brookes University, and Carol Komaromy, Lecturer in Health Studies, School of Health and Social Welfare, The Open University.

Chapter 8

Eric Brunner, Senior Lecturer in Epidemiology at University College London Medical School, and Harry Hemingway, Senior Lecturer in Epidemiology at University College London Medical School and Director of Research and Development at Kensington and Chelsea and Westminster Health Authority; at the Open University, Carol Komaromy, Lecturer, and Moyra Sidell, Senior Lecturer, both in the School of Health and Social Welfare, and Basiro Davey, Senior Lecturer in the Department of Biological Sciences.

Chapter 9

Mick Carpenter, Reader in Social Policy, University of Warwick, and Alan Dolan, Lecturer in Health and Social Studies, University of Warwick.

External assessors

Course assessor

Professor John Gabbay, Professor of Public Health Medicine, University of Southampton, and Director of the Wessex Institute for Health Research and Development.

Book 7 assessor

Professor James McEwen, Henry Mechan Chair of Public Health and Head of Department of Public Health, University of Glasgow.

Acknowledgements

The Course Team and the authors wish to thank the following people who, as contributors to previous editions of this book, made a lasting impact on the structure and philosophy of the present volume.

Nick Black, David Boswell, George Davey Smith, Alastair Gray, Robin Harding, Richard Holmes, Helen Lambert, Kevin McConway, Klim McPherson, Perry Morley, Stephen Pattison, Jennie Popay, Steven Rose, Clive Seale, Phil Strong, Steve Swithenby.

Cover images

Background: Nebulae in the Rho Ophiuchi region (Source: Anglo-Australian Observatory/Royal Observatory Edinburgh).

Middleground: Globe (Source: Mountain High Map™, Digital Wisdom, Inc).

Foreground: Patient entering a magnetic resonance imaging (MRI) scanner (Source: Willi and Deni McIntyre/ Science Photo Library)

The Open University Press, Celtic Court, 22 Ballmoor, Buckingham, MK18 1XW.

e-mail: enquiries@openup.co.uk

website: www.openup.co.uk

and

325 Chestnut Street, Philadelphia, PA 19106, USA.

First published 1985. Completely revised second edition published 1993.

This full-colour completely revised third edition published 2001.

A catalogue record of the book is available from the British Library.

Library of Congress Cataloging-in-Publication Data is available.

Edited, designed and typeset by The Open University.

Printed and bound in the United Kingdom by the Alden Group, Oxford.

ISBN 0335 20841X

This publication forms part of an Open University Level 2 course, U205 *Health and Disease*. The complete list of texts which make up this course can be found on the back cover. Details of this and other Open University courses can be obtained from the Call Centre, PO Box 724, The Open University, Milton Keynes MK7 6ZS, United Kingdom: tel. +44 (0)1908 653231, e-mail ces-gen@open.ac.uk

Alternatively, you may visit the Open University website at http://www.open.ac.uk where you can learn more about the wide range of courses and packs offered at all levels by The Open University.

3.1

CONTENTS

A note for the general reader

Dilemmas in UK Health Care considers a range of major and enduring dilemmas arising from the organisation and delivery of contemporary health care in the United Kingdom. The book analyses 'health care' in its widest possible sense, encompassing conventional health services, social and community services, disease-prevention and health-promotion initiatives and, finally, economic and fiscal policies that could have an impact on health. Throughout the book, we acknowledge the UK's reliance on informal carers as the principal mediators of health care in this country (as in others).

The book contains nine chapters, written by specialist authors whose academic affiliations are given in the study comment box at the start of each chapter.

Although the topics chosen for inclusion in the book are highly varied, each author has identified the principal dilemmas facing those involved in formulating policy, or delivering or receiving health care, and has analysed the reasons underlying the difficult and incompatible choices that may have to be made. In particular, the authors address the extent to which effective health care can be reconciled with efficiency in a cost-limited health-care system, while keeping in view the aim of distributing services equitably and delivering them humanely.

Chapter 1 serves as a general introduction to the themes of the book and sets the scene for the chapters to follow. Chapters 2 and 3 consider the structure and policy issues that shape the organisation of the NHS. Chapters 4, 5 and 6 focus on the experience of and expectations placed on formal and informal carers, and consider how these impact upon the quality of care that they give. Chapter 7 questions the extent to which technological solutions solve medical problems or create further dilemmas. Chapter 8 uses an extended case study on coronary heart disease to explore some of the key dilemmas in disease prevention. The debate is extended in Chapter 9 into the wider discussion of inequalities in health, and the dilemmas inherent in strategies for improving the nation's health by tackling poverty, inequality and social exclusion.

The book is fully indexed and referenced and contains a list of abbreviations and an annotated guide to further reading and to selected websites on the Internet. The list of further sources also includes details of how to access a regularly updated collection of Internet resources relevant to the *Health and Disease* series on a searchable database called ROUTES, which is maintained by The Open University. This resource is open to all readers of this book.

Dilemmas in UK Health Care is the seventh in a series of eight books on the subject of health and disease. The book is designed so that it can be read on its own, like any other textbook, or studied as part of U205 *Health and Disease*, a Level 2 course for Open University students. General readers do not need to make use of the study notes, learning objectives and other material inserted for OU students, although they may find these helpful. The text also contains references to a collection of previously published material and specially commissioned articles (*Health and Disease: A Reader*, Open University Press, 3rd edn 2001) prepared for the OU course: it is quite possible to follow the text without reading the articles referred to, although doing so will enhance your understanding of the contents of *Dilemmas in UK Health Care*.

Abbreviations used in this book

ACRE	Appropriateness of Coronary Revascularisation study
AIDS	acquired immune deficiency syndrome
BDA	British Dental Association
BMA	British Medical Association
BMI	body mass index
CABG	coronary artery bypass grafting
CAPD	continuous ambulatory peritoneal dialysis
CEPOD	confidential enquiries into peri-operative deaths
CHD	coronary heart disease
CHI	Commission for Health Improvement
CT	computer-aided tomography
DALY	disability-adjusted life-year
DSS	Department of Social Security
ECG	electrocardiogram
EN	Enrolled Nurse
FHS	Family Health Services
GDP	Gross Domestic Product
GMC	General Medical Council
GP	general practitioner
HBAI	households below average income
HCA	Health Care Assistant
HCHS	Hospital and Community Health Services
HDL	high-density lipoprotein
HFEA	Human Fertilisation and Embryology Authority
HIV	human immunodeficiency virus
HRT	hormone replacement therapy
ICT	information communication technology
ITU	intensive therapy unit
IVF	in vitro fertilisation
LDL	low-density lipoprotein
MDA	Medical Devices Agency
MI	myocardial infarction
MONICA	(international study) monitoring trends and determinants in cardiovascular disease
MRC	Medical Research Council
MRI	magnetic resonance imaging
MS	multiple sclerosis
NA	Nursing Auxiliary
NHS	National Health Service
NICE	National Institute for Clinical Excellence
NICU	neonatal intensive-care unit
NMR	nuclear magnetic resonance
NSF	National Service Framework
NTD	neural tube defect
NVQ	National Vocational Qualification
PAF	performance assessment framework
PAM	professions allied to medicine
PCG	Primary Care Group
PCT	Primary Care Trust
PD	peritoneal dialysis
PKU	phenylketonuria
PNMR	perinatal mortality rate
QALY	quality-adjusted life-year
R&D	research and development
RCN	Royal College of Nursing
RCT	randomised controlled trial
SMR	standardised mortality ratio
WHO	World Health Organisation

Study guide for OU students

(total of around 64 hours, including time for the TMA, spread over 4 weeks)

Chapter 1 is the shortest in the book, but the others are of relatively equal length. There are seven set Reader articles associated with this book for which you need to allow study time; we have also identified a number of *optional* articles recommended as enrichment of the themes explored in this book, if you have time. There is an audiotape called 'Who cares?' associated with Chapter 4 and a TV programme called 'Hospitals, who needs them?' which relates to Chapter 7.

1st week

Chapter 1	**Caring for life: dilemmas in health care**
Chapter 2	**Dilemmas in health care: responding to economic constraints**
Chapter 3	**Dilemmas in health-care management** Reader article by Ham (1999)

2nd week

Chapter 4	**Dilemmas in community care** Audiotape, 'Who cares?' optional Reader article by the Sainsbury Centre (1998)
Chapter 5	**Divisions in health-care labour** Reader articles by Davies (1995), and Doyal and Cameron (2001)
Chapter 6	**Evaluating health care: dilemmas posed by research and evidence** Reader article by Sackett *et al.* (1996) and three letters in reply; optional Reader article by Fitzpatrick and White (1997)

3rd week

Chapter 7	**Medical technology: solving problems or creating dilemmas?** Reader article by Alaszeswki and Harvey (2001); optional Reader article by Hardey (1999) TV programme 'Hospitals, who needs them?'
Chapter 8	**Preventing disease: the case of coronary heart disease** Reader article by Underwood and Bailey versus Shiu (1993); revise Reader article by Bowling (1999)

4th week

Chapter 9	**Poverty, inequality, social exclusion and health** Reader article by Gwatkin (2000); optional Reader article by Wilkinson (1996)

TMA completion

Dilemmas in UK Health Care continues the analysis of the UK health-care system, which began with the historical and comparative background to the present health service in *Caring for Health: History and Diversity* (Open University Press, 3rd edn 2001). It also builds on skills and concepts taught in other books in the Health and Disease series, principally those to do with data-interpretation, experimental methods, the demography and epidemiology of health and disease in the UK, and (to a limited degree) human biology and British culture. The structure of the book is briefly set out in 'A note for the general reader' (p.6), and is extensively developed in Chapter 1.

Study notes are given in a box at the start of each chapter. These primarily direct you to important links to other components of the course, such as the other books in the course series, the Reader, and audiovisual components. Major learning objectives are listed at the end of each chapter, along with questions that will enable you to check that you have achieved these objectives. The index includes key terms in orange type (also printed in bold in the text), which can be looked up easily as an aid to revision as the course proceeds. There is also a list of further sources for those who wish to pursue certain aspects of study beyond the scope of this book, either by consulting other books and articles or by logging on to specialist websites on the Internet.

The time allowed for studying *Dilemmas in UK Health Care* is four weeks, or about 64 hours. The schedule (left) gives a more detailed breakdown to help you to pace your study. You need not follow it rigidly, but try not to let yourself fall behind. If you find a section of the work difficult, do what you can at this stage, and then return to reconsider the material when you reach the end of the book.

There is a tutor-marked assignment (TMA) associated with this book; about 5 hours have been allowed for writing it up, *in addition to* the time spent studying the material that it assesses.

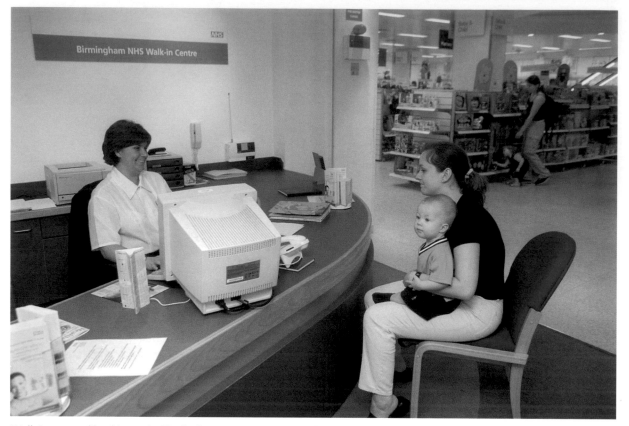

Walk-in centres like this one in Birmingham are nurse-run, readily accessible and an innovation in the NHS in the new millennium. They seem to offer a solution to some of the problems of overworked GPs and accident and emergency staff and make it easier for patients to get advice and treatment when they need it. But they raise several dilemmas. For example, will they help to cut treatment delays and reduce waiting lists or generate greater demands for health care? Will they promote patients' autonomy or damage their traditional cradle-to-grave relationship with a GP? How will they be evaluated and by what criteria? Dilemmas like these are debated in the chapters that follow. (Photo: John Harris/Report Digital)

C H A P T E R   1

Caring for life: dilemmas in health care

Study notes for OU students

This book focuses on the dilemmas that arise from the delivery of health care in the United Kingdom and particularly in the National Health Service. We assume that you understand the structure and funding of the NHS and the policy changes in its organisation between 1974 to 2001. These were introduced in Chapters 6, 7 and 9 of *Caring for Health: History and Diversity* (Open University Press, 3rd edn 2001). Here we build on the different meanings of health and disease and the status of medical knowledge, which were discussed in the first book in this series, *Medical Knowledge: Doubt and Certainty* (Open University Press, 2nd edn 1994; colour-enhanced 2nd edn 2001). This chapter was written by Carol Komaromy, Lecturer in Health Studies in the School of Health and Social Welfare at the Open University.

1.1   Universalising the best

One of the greatest challenges to health-care provision is to be able to meet health needs within the available resources, and to do this in a way that upholds the key principles of the National Health Service (NHS) in the United Kingdom, which have been in place since 1948. These state that health care:

- is universal;
- is free at the point of delivery, which means that people are not stigmatised by any need for charity; and finally,
- provides a good quality of service for everyone in need of health care.

These principles were summarised by Aneurin Bevan, the architect of the NHS, as 'universalising the best' and they continue to dominate the expectations of the NHS into the new millennium. However, trying to achieve them produces 'dilemmas'.

In this book, we use a distinct definition of **dilemmas**, that is: 'being forced to choose between less than ideal, even unpleasant alternatives.' In one sense, all dilemmas in health care are framed by ethical principles and many dilemmas in the UK are rooted therefore in the legacy of the founding principles and expectations of the NHS. This means that some of the dilemmas in health care are major and continuous, and apply to most settings. For example, how can the potentially endless health-care needs of everyone be met when the health-care budget is finite? Other dilemmas arise from specific types of care and are subject to change, such as the choice between different approaches to coronary heart disease, which you will read about in Chapter 8.

1.2   Broad and continuing health-care dilemmas

The rate of change in the NHS in the 1990s and the early part of the new millennium has been dramatic. The 'condition' of the NHS is an important voting issue, and, regardless of wider political changes and moves away from the 'ideology' of the welfare state, the NHS remains a central focus for UK citizens and continues to be valued by the majority of the population. Sustaining the key principles alongside these dramatic changes produces tensions that arise at different levels.

1.2.1 Ideological tensions in NHS care

The term **ideology** is used in this chapter to mean a doctrine that comprises a set of loosely linked ideas which serve to inform and justify action. For example, the ideology of 'individualism' holds that **autonomy**, as a means of expressing interests and fulfilling goals, is part of a whole set of individual freedoms which are held to be more important than those of 'the common good'. Making a service 'fit' the needs of individuals and ensuring that everyone gets the same high quality of care is one of the universal tasks of the NHS, and how governments facilitate this task also needs to be seen as being consistent with their particular political ideologies. Consequently, the demands of the NHS and the 'ideological correctness' of party politics have often been in conflict. This difficulty supports the view of the sociologist Stuart Hall (1985), that making these discordant elements of ideologies fit is part of the role of governments. One of the outcomes is that the shape of the NHS has changed according to the political policies of the different governments in power since 1948.

Regardless of government control, the size and range of NHS services make it difficult to consider as a coherent system of health care. Consequently, the tension between what happens at the centre at government level, and what happens at the periphery at the sites of care delivery, results in many dilemmas.

1.2.2 The structures of health care

The policies and principles of the NHS are examples of **social structures** which frame the way in which health care is delivered. These structures might be open and flexible, or conversely, rigid and resistant to change. Recognising structures in society will help you to consider the extent to which they have been produced by social and political forces and the extent to which they can be changed. For example, structures such as health and economic policies are socially produced and likely to change over time, whereas others, such as the age- or sex-structure of the UK population, are 'given' and therefore unlikely to change — at least in the short to medium term.

● What are some of the effects of demographic change on the delivery of UK health care?

■ The health needs of people tend to increase with age and many of the demands for health care in the NHS are from older people. This has raised the problem of who should provide that care when there is a comparatively smaller population of younger people able to serve as carers. It also tips the balance of financial contributions when there are more demands on fewer people to contribute national insurance payments for health care.

The political and economic dilemmas of care provision will change according to the demands of society, but there are ethical principles underpinning health and social care.

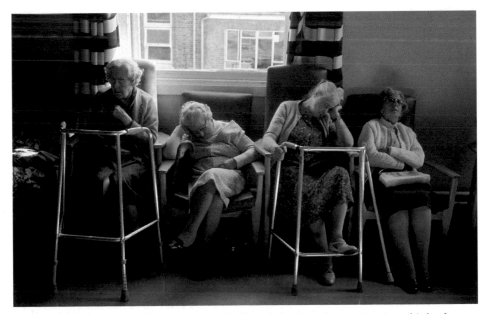

Despite the move to institutional care provided largely by the private sector, two-thirds of hospital beds in England and Wales are occupied by people over 65 years old (Ferriman, 2000). This nursing home in the Midlands provides care for people who would previously have been cared for in a geriatric hospital ward. (Photo: Michael Abrahams/Network)

1.2.3 What kind of health service?

Ethical problems in health care arise at different levels. For example, there is an economic assumption on the part of governments of all political persuasions that the resources from which health care is provided *should* be limited. From an ethical point of view, this 'rationing' is harder to defend. Furthermore, what these limits are and how they are set is debated and decided in the wider political arena, but they depend upon how health is defined and this is also an ethical concern.

The concept of **health** is broad and ranges from the 'absence of disease' at one end of the spectrum to 'a state of complete physical, mental and social well-being' at the other end, as defined by the World Health Organisation (WHO) declaration of 1946. This raises the question of what sort of health care a national health service can provide. Along the health continuum, health care can mean the treatment of sick people, the prevention of disease or the promotion of health, with care-givers being anyone from a range of formal and informal carers and in many different settings. The analogy of the 'stream of ill-health' is often used to illustrate the health continuum and to make the point that it is better to prevent people falling into the 'river' than it is to have to rescue them from drowning or even resuscitate them. For example, the NHS acute sector of care has most often been focused 'downstream' on treatments provided by acute hospitals, and it is not surprising, therefore, that despite its requirement to provide health care, the NHS has often been accused of providing a sickness service — treating disease rather than promoting health. This remains an ongoing debate, and one which recurs throughout this book.

Therefore, health care is not just about making sound clinical judgements — it is also subject to issues that would seem to be unrelated to 'health', but which are crucial aspects of health-care decision-making. An understanding of health decisions requires an understanding of the way that health is politically, economically, ideologically and ethically framed as much as a knowledge of the detail that arises at the level of health-care delivery. The following case study provides an illustration of these wider issues.

1.3 Neonatal intensive-care needs: a case study

In September 2000, the findings of a research study published in the *British Medical Journal* and entitled 'National census of availability of neonatal intensive-care' achieved headline status (Parmanum *et al.*, 2000). The study was conducted in response to concerns that the supply of neonatal cots did not match demand and that the allocation of this type of care provision had changed from an 'efficient use of resources' to crisis management (p. 727).

1.3.1 Background

Within the western world, the focus has shifted from maternal mortality as an indicator of the nation's health to **perinatal mortality**. The perinatal mortality rate is the number of babies born dead after 24 weeks' gestation (stillbirths) or dying in the first week of life, per 1000 total (live and still) births. Selecting this form of mortality as 'avoidable' means that neonatal intensive-care units (NICUs) have become the showcases of the capacity of modern medicine and there has been a sharp rise in technological advances in this area.

This rise in profile was reinforced by the Winterton Report (House of Commons Health Committee, 1991–2), which acknowledged that the outcome for very-low-birthweight babies was better if they were treated in **tertiary centres**. These centres provide services, usually accessed in the first instance by referral from consultant medical staff, for patients with complex or rare conditions, and serving a geographical area and population base wider than a single health authority. A report that followed the Winterton Report, called *Children First* (Department of Health, 1993), compared the 52 per cent survival rate of babies in NICUs in tertiary centres with 22 per cent in NICUs in acute hospitals (secondary centres). The report also identified the economies of scale that larger units make, emphasising that it was cheaper to nurse a baby who needed full ventilatory support in a large unit than in a smaller one. (At that time, the cost of care for a baby in supported ventilation was quoted as £450 per day in a large centre compared to £640 in a smaller one.)

The recommendation from both reports was that babies in need of neonatal intensive care should be transferred to tertiary centres. In reality, this means that where it is possible to predict early or high-risk birth, then the mother and baby will be transferred to the tertiary centre before the birth. This is called an *in utero* transfer.

Neonatal intensive care is an example of a high-cost, low-provision form of care. Low-birthweight infants account for only 7 per cent of all births, but between 50 and 80 per cent of all perinatal deaths. The care in NICUs is dependent upon specialised technological devices including neonatal ventilators and monitoring equipment, multidisciplinary teams of specialised staff including support services of all types, and a specialised environment, including incubators and premises that can accommodate specialised equipment, staff and parents. It follows that high levels of specialised resources are required to provide this type of care.

In many instances, the care that is being provided is replacing the function of the uterus of the infants' biological mother, since two-thirds of the babies who are treated in NICUs are **pre-term infants**, that is they are born before 36 weeks' gestation. There is a direct correlation between the degree of prematurity and the intensity of the care that is needed. For example, an infant born at 24 weeks' gestation will require continuous support, whereas an infant of 35 weeks' gestation will require considerably less service than a tertiary centre offers.

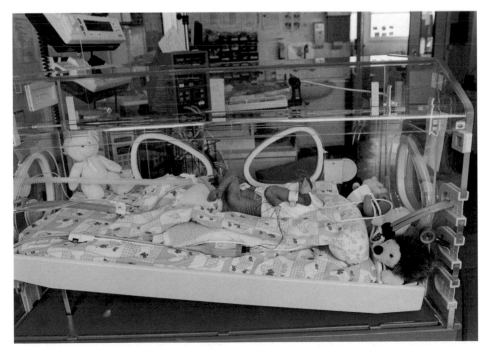

Neonatal intensive-care units (NICUs) are dependent upon highly qualified staff with specialist skills, both in the use of sophisticated equipment and interpersonal skills for parental support. Working in NICUs is an extremely stressful occupation. (Photo: Mike Levers)

1.3.2 Neonatal intensive-care availability

The study by Parmanum and colleagues (2000) into the availability of neonatal intensive care in the UK was conducted over a three-month period from 1 April to 30 June 1999 and involved the 37 largest NICUs accepting high-risk babies in the UK. In other words, these are the centres to which babies in need of intensive care should be sent in order for them to receive the 'best' care. The study did not include mothers and infants in need of specialist care not available at that hospital. For example, there are very few tertiary centres in which a form of lung by-pass treatment is available, the treatment used for babies who have inhaled meconium (faeces) prior to delivery. Likewise, not all tertiary centres offer neonatal surgery.

There were 382 babies recorded in the study altogether, of which 65 births (138 babies) were multiple. In the three months of the study, 309 babies were transferred from their local health service to a tertiary centre; of these, 264 were *in utero* and 45 were transferred post-natally. The main reason for *in utero* transfer (in 245 of the 264 transferred babies) was a lack of available NICU cots in the maternity units to which the women in labour were admitted. On nine of the occasions, the reason given for lack of a cot was a shortage of staff.

While being able to universalise the best is dependent upon adequate resources, this example raises a dilemma of how to allocate neonatal intensive care to those babies who need it *at the time of need* when there are not enough cots available.

● Why might it be important to include 'time of need' in this statement?

■ This is a different issue from there being enough cots available over a period of time, because demands within any period will fluctuate. While the birth rate is summarised to provide a monthly or annual rate, the timing of 'at risk' births is irregular and unpredictable.

Thus, while it is possible to make economies of scale, in reality there needs to be some spare capacity to cope with emergencies. There are all sorts of reasons why planning emergency care is difficult, and caring for babies at a distance from their home environment can add to the problems.

Findings from the study

The research team set out to measure the 'adequacy of the service' against 'existing national recommendations regarding good practice' and concluded that 'breaches of these recommendations were commonplace.' The authors discussed the implications of these results and included a plea that the meaning of a neonatal intensive-care cot should include 'not just a bed space but also the equipment and staff that allow that space to be utilised for intensive care' (Parnamum *et al.*, 2000, p. 728). Furthermore, although the long-term outcome effects of transfer were not measured, the researchers concluded that 'the psychological and financial burdens placed on families involved in any type of transfer are without a doubt considerable' (p. 729).

1.3.3 Dilemmas in neonatal transfers

● What immediate dilemma are parents of babies who are transferred to tertiary centres likely to face?

■   Parents have to choose between wanting the best for their babies but possibly at the cost of not being close to them, and consequently suffer the damage that separation might bring to everyone involved.

However, the greater dilemma might be for the parents of those babies who stay in smaller units with what is considered to be sub-optimal care, and the potential consequences that arise from this in terms of possible disability.

●   Beyond the issues about resource availability, suggest what ethical dilemma this case study raises.

■   Long-term care falls mostly into the domain of the parents of infants. They receive various degrees of support (an issue discussed in Chapter 4). Of course, there is no way of knowing for certain when any damage may have occurred, and parents are often left speculating about possible causes of any disability.

The plight of very small and fragile infants is likely to capture public sympathy in a way that it is difficult for governments to ignore. Publicising medical crises is one way of pressurising governments into taking action and when the report was published it reflected on the political policy decisions about providing NHS care and threatened to tarnish the high-profile showcases of neonatal medicine. This example also highlights the sympathy given to small babies, which is much greater than for other groups in society who are less appealing. When there is competition for resources these 'appeal' factors can play a major part. Politicians have to manage these tensions when they become public issues and make difficult and sometimes unpopular choices.

What at first sight appears to be a simple economic problem of insufficient resources is in fact much more than that, and further dilemmas can be drawn from the study. There is an assumption that providing adequate resources for neonatal care could solve the problems associated with premature birth, but this is not necessarily the case.

The clinical evidence on NICU treatment has focused on *mortality* outcomes, but the evidence on *morbidity* is patchy and poorly collated. The *Children First* report highlighted the potential for adverse outcomes of cerebral palsy, developmental delay, poor vision and hearing, epilepsy and loss of limbs in 'rescued' babies born prematurely. Should the focus of health-care resources be on treatment rather than on prevention of premature birth, when there is so little evidence on clinical outcomes and long-term problems? This raises the question of whether enough resources are devoted to preserving the pregnancy and preventing premature birth.

It is also relevant that perinatal mortality, congenital malformation and low birth-weight are all greater in social classes IV and V, virtually whatever dataset is examined. It could be argued that using 'rescue medicine' to solve immediate problems not only continues to ignore the causes of prematurity and low birth-weight, but also reinforces the perceived power of neonatal doctors who are at the leading edge of medical technology.

●   What clinical dilemma does this raise?

■   The clinical dilemma of whether or not it is better to attempt to 'cure' premature birth when so little is known about the outcomes and the causes. Preventing premature births might be outside the domain of health care, as the evidence suggests a link to social causes of premature birth.

Thus, dilemmas are confounded by concerns about the sanctity of life, which at first sight appears to be an entirely 'ethical' consideration in the domain of clinicians and medical ethicists, but which also involves the state and society in deciding what resources should be allocated to whom.

This short case study has served to highlight some of the dilemmas in UK health care for the new millennium. It illustrates how wider issues, which provide the context for health care, are interdependent; not only do these wider aspects frame decisions about the provision of health services, but they also interact in ways that produce further complexity and new dilemmas. These dilemmas at the political, ideological, ethical, clinical and personal level set the scene for the rest of this book.

1.4   Introduction to Chapters 2 to 9

Each of the following chapters takes a particular topic of interest in UK health care and examines it from the point of view of the problems it raises. We have tried to focus on key dilemmas, each of which is framed by wider political, economic, ideological and ethical issues. For example, while the social structures of health care are dynamic and changing, the need to provide 'the best' is enduring.

In writing this book, we aim to give you an understanding of the key dilemmas at the time of writing and also to equip you with the skills to be able to analyse future changes. The analysis in each of the chapters is quite detailed and is written by a specialist in that area. Therefore, as you read through the remaining chapters, you might find it useful to use the above themes to help you to frame your study. This is a device for getting some purchase on what are quite complex and detailed areas of health care. Furthermore, keeping in mind broader structural issues will also help you to retain a critical approach to the study of dilemmas in UK health care.

Chapter 2, 'Dilemmas in health care: responding to economic constraints', focuses on how economic decisions are made in the NHS and considers the principles within which the NHS deals with limited resources. The main form of health-care allocation is made according to a system of rationing but, as the chapter argues, this takes many forms and each method carries its own costs. This discussion of the dilemmas in economics and the NHS system of health care sets the scene for the key concern of how to manage its size and diversity while affording a universal service — the subject of Chapter 3, 'Dilemmas in health-care management'. The 'managerialism' of the 1980s has left a legacy of power tensions between clinical autonomy and the need for greater control of the NHS as a public service and resource. The key dilemma seems to be that governments need to devolve power from the centre to the peripheries where health care is delivered, while at the same time staying in control of the economic and political agendas. When clinicians are also in the role of managing the demand and supply of services, dilemmas are produced at all levels of health care.

Health and social care are brought together in Chapter 4, 'Dilemmas in community care', which considers the dilemmas that arise from the shift to community care and how far the needs of people in the community have been met. In particular, the chapter asks how much of community care is dependent upon informal carers and the extent to which they are exploited, despite the more formal recognition of their role in the policies of the 1990s. The chapter also considers the extent to which advocacy can solve the dilemmas that arise from the relative powerlessness of certain groups in receipt of community care. Chapter 5, 'Divisions in health-care labour', shifts the focus from informal to formal carers, and considers the professionals who work in the NHS and the dilemmas that arise from divisions of labour as a form of management. It uses a case study of the role of health-care assistants in the NHS to illustrate the strategies that employers use to manage the tension between efficiency and *equity* — the provision of services according to need.

Providing good-quality care to all in need is one way of meeting the ethical demand of equity and quality, but evaluation of what is good quality is beset with dilemmas. Chapter 6, 'Evaluating health care: dilemmas posed by research and evidence', addresses some of these dilemmas and asks what counts as evidence in evidence-based health care. It raises concerns about how to choose the best type of evaluation, how to put this evidence into practice and how to involve patients in decisions when they might use different criteria from that of clinical effectiveness. Much of health-care evaluation is focused on new types of care, and health-care innovations are seen as both the solution to health problems and the cause of the escalating cost of health care. Chapter 7, 'Medical technology: solving problems or creating dilemmas?', raises the dilemmas that arise from technological innovations by focusing on three specific case studies: magnetic resonance imaging, renal dialysis and 'e' health — the use of electronic communication technology in health care. These case studies also raise issues about the shift of expertise to patients and the role of the acute hospital in the new millennium.

In Chapter 8, 'Preventing disease: the case of CHD', we ask whether or not prevention is better than cure by applying this question to the case study of coronary heart disease (CHD). This detailed exploration of a multifactorial disease illustrates some of the complexity within disease prevention, screening and treatment decisions. The relationship between heart disease and social inequalities questions the role of health care in CHD reduction. The suggestion that the NHS is a 'sickness' and not a 'health' service is picked up in the final chapter, Chapter 9, 'Poverty, inequality, social exclusion and health', which brings this book to a close. It asks whether we should give greater priority to measures aimed at reducing poverty or economic inequality in the expectation that this strategy will be more effective in reducing the incidence of ill health and disease than will even greater expenditure on health care. Finally, the consequences of any policies that attempt to reduce inequalities produce dilemmas not just in terms of economics, but also in terms of justice.

1.4.1 A note about the authors

In this book, we have been careful not to take sides when competing options are being discussed; our aim has been to reveal the *nature* of the dilemmas — not to offer solutions. The chapters that follow have been written by specialists in certain areas of health policy or health-care research, mostly from educational or research institutions outside the Open University. The editor of this book has not attempted to disguise the somewhat different 'voices' expressed in each chapter, but you should be aware of who the authors are and where their interests and priorities may therefore lie. This information is given at the start of each chapter, in the box containing study notes for Open University students.

OBJECTIVES FOR CHAPTER 1

When you have completed this chapter, you should be able to:

1.1 Define and use, or recognise definitions and applications of, each of the terms printed in **bold** in the text.

1.2 Recognise and distinguish between the wider influences on dilemmas in health-care decision making.

1.3 Discuss the complexity of responding to health-care needs within limited resources.

QUESTIONS FOR CHAPTER 1

1 (*Objective 1.2*)

Use the example of the shortage of neonatal care cots in tertiary centres to discuss what further dilemmas might be raised by political solutions.

2 (*Objective 1.3*)

Is it safe to assume that *all premature* babies would benefit from neonatal intensive care? Use the case study to suggest the potential problems that arise from this question.

CHAPTER 2

Dilemmas in health care: responding to economic constraints

Study notes for OU students

Chapter 9 of *Caring for Health: History and Diversity* (Open University Press, 3rd edition 2001), introduced you to international patterns of health-care funding and provision. This chapter extends those ideas into a focused discussion of how economic constraints impact upon health care in the NHS in the UK and the consequent dilemmas. This chapter was written by Alan Williams, who is Professor of Economics, Centre for Health Economics at the University of York.

2.1   Economics and health care

The two broad objectives of the NHS are to improve the health of the whole population, and to reduce inequalities in people's lifetime experience of health as much as possible, given the resource constraints that the system faces. All public services face budget constraints, and the NHS is no exception. The appropriate level at which to set those resource constraints is, of course, arguable, but this chapter is concerned primarily with the *principles* within which the NHS deals with economic constraints, rather than the absolute level of funding. As you will see, these principles are often in conflict — creating dilemmas for policy-makers, individual health-care staff (particularly doctors) and service users.

The NHS was set up in 1948 to replace the setting of priorities according to willingness and ability to pay with the setting of priorities according to **need** (defined here as 'capacity to benefit from health care').

● Outline the main reason why this change of priorities was made.

■ The perceived problem was that opportunities to improve the health of poorer people were being neglected relative to looking after the health of the better off.[1]

For example, **rationing** is a process for ensuring that everyone gets their appropriate share of some scarce good, in this case health care. There is nothing intrinsically good or bad about rationing, but one could argue whether one way of doing it is better or worse than another way. The NHS cannot abolish the need for rationing, because to do so it would have to abolish scarcity, and that is beyond the bounds of feasibility. But although rationing is inevitable, we have some choice over what *principles* should govern it, or, in other words, what set of priorities it should reflect. So the ethics of rationing are really the ethics of different principles for rationing. To be ethically defensible, these principles must reflect the objectives of the NHS and assist in achieving them (New, 1997).

Historically, the management of resources, and the setting of priorities, was largely in the hands of the medical profession and was seen as part of their management responsibilities as clinicians. This role, however, came increasingly under challenge during the 1970s, and with the advent of the internal market in the 1990s a great deal of the power previously exercised by doctors was transferred to managers. In the process, the rationing dilemmas which doctors had previously wrestled with in private were discussed in a much more public domain, and even became the stuff of television drama.

2.2   The internal market of the NHS

2.2.1   The purchaser–provider split

In the late 1980s and early 1990s, the NHS underwent the most radical overhaul in its 40-year history, intended to put in place more effective mechanisms for delivering health care more equitably within cost constraints. An **internal market** or 'quasi-market' in health care was created. The reason for this guarded terminology is that

[1] *Caring for Health: History and Diversity* (Open University Press, 3rd edn 2001), Chapter 6.

these markets do not place purchasing power in the hands of patients (or their private insurers), as in an ordinary market for private health care. Instead, purchasing power is placed in the hands of public authorities charged with exercising the purchasing (or demand) function on behalf of patients generally. Purchasing authorities were given the task of estimating the service needs for their locality, and they bought these services using funds allocated by central government. The health-care providers — NHS Trusts, such as acute hospitals, mental health services, ambulance services, etc. — tendered for contracts from the purchasers in a competitive market, each Trust *in theory* bidding against other providers of equivalent services in their locality — including those in the private sector. The separation of supply and demand sides of this market was dubbed the **purchaser–provider split**.

In this way it was hoped to gain the advantages of 'real' markets without the disadvantages. The chief *disadvantage* of ordinary markets is that the distribution of purchasing power does not match the distribution of the need for health care.

2.2.2 A market without prices

In the internal market of the NHS, the two independent influences of demand and supply have to be reconciled. In an ordinary market, this is achieved by *price* adjustments. According to market principles therefore, if demand exceeds supply, prices should rise until the two are brought into balance, or equilibrium; otherwise, queues form and/or people go away empty-handed. Conversely, if supply exceeds demand, prices should fall until the two are brought into balance; otherwise, unsold stocks pile up which could have been cleared by price reductions. But what is to happen when we decide to do away with prices — as in the NHS?

The chief *advantage* of markets is that they decentralise decision-making, thus reducing the information overload on central planners. There is no way in which the treatment decisions made for every patient can be submitted to some central authority for approval before they are carried out. So health-care systems have to find ways in which those with the relevant local knowledge and expertise use it to make a limited set of decisions about 'who gets what', which then interacts with the equally limited decisions made centrally by others about what can be prescribed. The system as a whole is supposed to operate cohesively. The design, and redesign, of health-care systems can be seen as a constant search for this ideal.

The purchasing authorities only need to know about how beneficial the different health-care activities are to patients, and compare the benefits with the prices that the providers will charge (just as consumers have to do when shopping). They do not need to know anything about the production process or how efficient it is, but they do need to know something about the quality of the product they are buying.

The providing authorities, on the other hand, only need to know how best to organise the supply of health-care activities and to find ways of doing so that fall within the price that the purchasers are willing to pay. Prices will be negotiated and play an equilibrating role once more. Competition between providers will keep them efficient (or they lose out to rivals who can provide better products at lower prices). Unfortunately, this neat solution at the level of principle does not work too smoothly in practice for reasons that will be discussed next.

2.2.3 Dilemmas in the health-care market

In the first place, distributing resources according to some centrally determined notion of need does not guarantee that they will be *used* in accordance with that centrally determined notion. Indeed, the whole point of the internal market was to provide some local discretion for purchasers to act in accordance with local circumstances. So here is a dilemma, encapsulated in simultaneous demands for more local discretion but less postcode rationing!

Secondly, the role of GPs remains ambiguous in that they both provide primary-care services to their patients, and purchase secondary and tertiary services from hospitals and other providers — so they are on *both* sides of the supply-and-demand division at the heart of the internal market. There is potentially a conflict of interest between what is good for them as providers and what is good for their patients for whom they are acting as purchasers.

Thirdly, the purchaser–provider split exposed how little was known about both the costs and the benefits of most health-care activities. The information required to make a market work properly was simply not available. Moreover, much of the information that the purchasers needed (e.g. on the benefits of treatments) was in the hands of providers, who had strong motivation to use it selectively.

Fourthly, in many communities there is only one hospital that is readily accessible, so that realistic competition in the provision of hospital care is impossible. There are also specialist centres of excellence to which patients might be referred. To overcome this problem, the central authority has to act as a regulator, collecting data on prices and costs and checking that monopoly power is not being abused.

Fifthly, because the viability of providers (mainly hospitals) depends on the winning of contracts, which are negotiated with purchasers by managers, this has generated a shift of power from hospital consultants to hospital managers, which the doctors greatly resent. Moreover, this has came on top of a shift of power from hospital consultants to GPs due to the role of GPs in the purchasing authorities. It is hardly surprising therefore that it is hospital consultants who are the most disaffected group over the 'internal market' reforms in the NHS. Although the terminology changed when the new Labour government took over in 1997 — preferring the language of 'integrated care' and a 'seamless service' — the fundamental notion of a purchaser–provider split remains, and there appears to be little likelihood of a return to the previous supplier-dominated regime.

Despite the appeal of the internal market, the problems associated with making choices about how to prioritise health care needs remain.

2.3 Rationing by waiting lists

When health care is rationed according to willingness and ability to pay, there is no need for waiting lists. Those who are still saving up to buy treatments they cannot at present afford are not on anybody's list! However, when health care is rationed by need, someone has to divide people into categories according to the extent and urgency of their needs. Some people get immediate treatment, some people have to wait for a while, and some get nothing. The people who are waiting for a while get onto a list, and although they are a minority of all NHS patients, they attract a great deal of attention, because people have come to regard NHS waiting lists as a sign of failure or badge of shame.

It could be argued that waiting lists are an essential feature of a sensibly run system. Apart from accidents and emergencies, which go immediately into the hospital sector, the first point of contact with the system for most NHS patients will be with their GP in the primary care sector. In the vast majority of such cases, the patient is treated there and then by the GP (though they may have had to wait for an appointment). In a few cases, the GP may decide that the matter is too urgent or too difficult to handle in primary care and will refer the patient to a hospital doctor.

The GP is using a **triage system** of prioritising patients for hospital treatment, which has three categories of 'urgent', 'soon' and 'routine'. This categorisation affects the patient's position on the waiting list and the period within which a hospital appointment is allocated. The 'routine' category is the one that has attracted the most attention, because for such patients there may be a wait of weeks or usually months for the initial outpatient consultation. When this eventually arrives the patient may be treated on the spot, and/or referred back to the GP for treatment, and/or offered inpatient treatment for which, once more, there may be varying lengths of waiting time according to the urgency or seriousness of the case, and the pressure on local resources. The amount of capacity available for the more routine cases will vary from day to day, and from week to week according to the fluctuations in the urgent work, *unless* the system runs continuously with a lot of spare capacity, which would be very costly.

● Waiting lists are highly visible representations of a rationed resource, but what features make them appear to be a sign of failure or underfunding?

■ Two phenomena are typically highlighted: the growing number of people on NHS waiting lists; and the long time that some people have to wait.

2.3.1 Handling waiting lists

Paradoxically, as the capacity of the NHS increases, the number of people waiting for treatment also tends to increase, and there is nothing inherently bad about this phenomenon in itself. The reason for this apparently shocking statement can most easily be seen by imagining, for example, that each hospital consultant has a constant number of patients waiting for treatment. In that case, the more consultants there are, the more people there will be on waiting lists. Moreover, getting more people onto waiting lists would be quite consistent with a decline in waiting *times*, if each consultant maintained a constant flow of new attenders but saw more of them each week. So there is no reason why more people waiting should in itself be a bad thing. It will depend on what is happening to the 'flows', rather than what is the size of the 'stock'. There are many other NHS professionals with waiting lists and the principle applies to them all equally

The length of time that people have to wait is of far more interest to individual patients than the number of people waiting. Here it is important to distinguish average waiting times from the maximum. The latter is often cited as if it were the norm, when it is actually the experience of only a few. But there is an interesting balancing act to be done here between the wait for the initial outpatient appointment and the wait for any subsequent inpatient treatment that may be required. There is then not one queue, but several different queues, which vary according to demand. It is not obvious which is the more important for the individual patient — the delay in finding out what is wrong and what might be done about it, or the delay in any treatment that may be required (given that urgent treatment will usually be given quickly).

Waiting lists are an intrinsic part of the priority-setting mechanisms of the NHS, and they play a key role in ensuring that the more urgent and important cases are dealt with first. However, the following questions would provide the basis for an appraisal of this mechanism by NHS staff.

1   Are the right criteria being used to place people on the waiting list?

2   Are the right criteria being used to control who gets priority once on the waiting list?

3   Do the specialists who manage NHS waiting lists have the appropriate incentives to keep waiting list numbers down to manageable levels?

4   Do the managers have appropriate incentives to sustain capacity at a level that is optimal for the citizenry both as potential patients and as taxpayers?

In July 2001, a report on inpatient and outpatient waiting times in the NHS revealed that waiting lists and waiting times were considered to be too long for many patients. The report also cited 'large geographical inequalities'. Incentives to reduce waiting lists include additional funding to NHS Trusts, best practice guidelines and a task force to 'identify solutions' for individual Trusts (Department of Health, 2001a).

Although there is an increasing degree of representation of patients in decision-making forums including the National Patient Access Team, who will be included in initiatives to reduce waiting lists, a large *democratic* deficit remains. In the NHS structures of 2001 there is no place for local accountability since the only direct route is through parliament.

2.3.2 The costs of waiting for treatment

Elective surgery is the segment of medical practice where the ideological conflict between two entirely different methods of priority setting for health care is played out most obviously and dramatically — that is, priority setting by willingness and ability to pay, and priority setting by need. However, even within the latter method there is yet another priority-setting issue to be faced — namely who should get priority in being selected for treatment once they are on a waiting list? One obvious principle is first come–first served.

● What is the main disadvantage of prioritising in this way?

■ People awaiting treatments that would bring about big health gains would be kept waiting because there may be large numbers of people awaiting smaller health improvements ahead of them in the queue.

Another rule might be that no-one should wait longer than some pre-specified time. This again gives precedence to length of wait no matter how large or small the health gains, and has the additional side-effect that one way to avoid running into the limit is to offer treatment to fewer people in the first place. Some complex systems make the length of wait inversely proportional to the expected benefits, so that patients awaiting major gains wait a short time, while those awaiting minor gains wait much longer.

In money terms, it may look efficient to keep patients waiting for hours for appointments, rather than 'waste' the time of the NHS's employees who are not being fully occupied; but since people's time could well be used doing other things that they value, this financial saving is bought at a high cost to patients! This dilemma provides the clue as to why economists insist that the proper concept to use here is

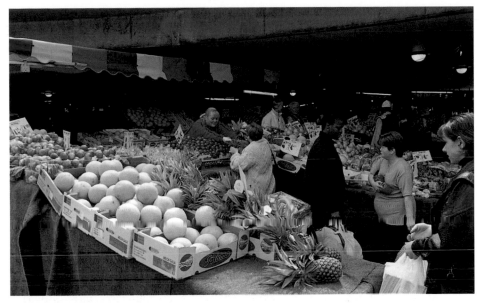

People who shop for goods directly can choose whether they want to wait for what they purchase. (Photo: Mike Levers)

that of **opportunity cost**, which says that the value of any resource is the most valuable *alternative* use to which the resource might have been put. This does not depend on money changing hands at all, although in a market, where people compete for a resource, its eventual price will be a good indicator of the opportunity cost of that resource. There is no market for resources such as patients' time, so we have no easy way of calculating its value, but we do know that its value is not zero!

The dilemmas that waiting lists produce are experienced most acutely at the levels of consultation between health-care professionals (most often doctors) and patients. GPs as the gatekeepers and key purchasers of health care are the front line decision-makers and particularly concerned to reduce waiting times.

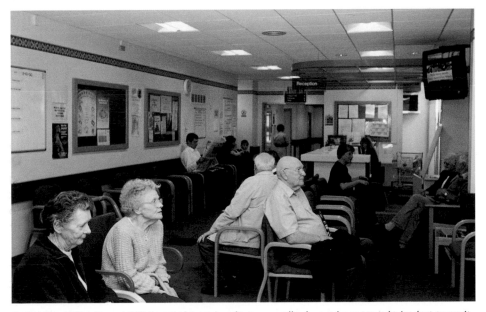

Patients waiting in an NHS hospital to see a doctor usually do not have any choice but to wait. (Photo: Mike Levers)

2.4 Rationing: individual treatments

At a fundamental level, patients do not come to health-care professionals demanding health care, but demanding better *health* according to their individual perceptions of health. The task of the health professional is then to work out what (if any) health care would in fact be most likely to produce an improvement in health for that particular individual, and to organise its provision. But they are limited in their ability to do this by their own knowledge and skills and by the resources at their disposal (including their own time and energy). Therefore, they have to weigh up how much of these limited resources it is worth investing in each particular patient, and they are likely to do this by assessing how much benefit will result.

This is what **prioritising according to need** means, and it requires a comparative judgement to be made as to whose needs are greatest. Consequently, it involves an inescapable inter-personal judgement, which goes beyond deciding what is best for any one individual. The more stringent are the available resources (for example, the more the doctor is short of time), the more stringent will be the criteria for deciding who gets what. It is at this informal and narrowly focused level that implicit notions of **cost-effectiveness** have always been a pervasive feature of clinical practice, and what has slowly emerged is the need to apply such thinking explicitly and systematically to a much wider range of phenomena than face-to-face interaction between doctors and patients.

Rationing occurs when, because of resource constraints, a treatment is withheld which the doctor believes will benefit the patient, but also because the doctor believes that the saved resources would do more good if devoted to somebody else. There are many reasons for believing that resources can be used more effectively, and these include examples of age, complex clinical issues and lifestyle.

- Read through the case studies A, B and C in Box 2.1. According to the above definition of rationing, in which of the three cases has rationing occurred?

- Case A — yes, by withholding the more expensive antibiotic and trying to save resources.

  Case B — yes, by trying to maximise the good and choosing the woman with dependent children.

  Case C — no, because the decision rests on the doctor's view that the treatment is not in the best interests of the patient, despite what the patient thinks.

- Now read Case D in Box 2.1 and make a note of what further information you would require, in order to decide whether rationing has occurred.

- In this case it is unclear whether or not rationing has occurred, because we know nothing about the relative cost-effectiveness of the two drugs, or the second doctor's reasons for switching to it. 'Newer' does not necessarily mean more cost-effective, or more clinically effective.

The main claim to the drug's **efficacy**, i.e. its clinical effectiveness, may rest on trials that did not include people like this patient. Older people are usually suffering from several different conditions, and hence are excluded from many clinical trials because they make the results less clear-cut!

Rationing individual treatments assumes that doctors work in neutral environments, whereas in reality they are subject to a range of other influences on their decision-making.

Box 2.1   Case studies of rationing individual treatments

Case A

A patient is diagnosed as having a urinary-tract infection, and is prescribed an antibiotic which cures 90 per cent of such cases quite quickly. The doctor knows that, for the cases for which this treatment does not work, he or she can fall back on a much more expensive antibiotic with an even higher cure rate and a lower risk of adverse side-effects.

Case B

A kidney becomes available for transplantation, and from the waiting list are selected two patients who pass the tissue-matching tests that indicate whether or not such a transplantation is likely to be successful. On purely clinical grounds there is no basis for choosing between them. However, the transplant centre has a policy, endorsed by a lay panel, which results in priority being given to a woman aged 30 with two school-age children, over a woman aged 45 whose children have left home.

Case C

A patient requests a screening test which is known to have rather dangerous side-effects and so is normally offered only to high-risk patients for whom the benefits are likely to outweigh the risks. The patient is not in that category and is consequently refused the test. He eventually finds a doctor abroad who will carry out the test, which is rather expensive, and in addition to the medical fees he has to pay his travel and accommodation costs, all of which he meets out of his own pocket.

Case D

An older patient is diagnosed as having rather high blood pressure, for which his GP prescribes a tried and trusted drug that he has been relying on for years. A few weeks later the patient returns with an unrelated condition, and sees a different GP that day, who notices which anti-hypertensive drug (to reduce blood pressure) the patient is on. After assuring herself that the drug is in fact working, she nevertheless suggests switching to a different and more up-to-date drug which came onto the market only recently and which, she explains, 'is becoming more widely used all the time'. Was the first GP rationing?

2.5   Incentives and individual dilemmas for NHS doctors

Doctors inevitably face conflicts of interest in choosing between priorities such as:

- the treatment of current patients;
- improving their knowledge for the benefit of their own future patients;
- engaging in research, and in the training of other doctors, for the benefit of other people's future patients;
- managing their own practice;
- satisfying their responsibilities towards their personal dependants;
- fulfilling themselves!

These tensions can be seen as an optimisation problem requiring the consideration of costs and benefits, but it can also be seen as an *incentive* problem. What are the relative pecuniary and non-pecuniary rewards of each activity? To the extent that money matters (and it usually matters to some extent), how does the remuneration system for doctors affect their behaviour? The interaction between the annual salary structure of NHS pay and the fee-for-service structure of private-sector pay inevitably affects the balance between NHS and private work for hospital consultants. Giving a GP a drug budget inevitably affects his or her prescribing behaviour.

It can be said that some GPs are perhaps more likely to undertake postgraduate education or engage in research if they are specifically paid to do so. For example, the postgraduate education allowance is only paid to those GPs who participate in activities that are sanctioned as being part of continuing education. All of these things will interact with their supposed duty to do the best for each patient, no matter what the costs.

The dilemmas in health care start at this individual level, although most of the public discussion has focused on the way in which they surface at a much higher level of policy and practice.

If key people are offered **perverse incentives** — which include a shift of costs onto others rather than improving overall efficiency, or promoting private practice instead of making the NHS work better — then it will prove to be very difficult to justify pouring more resources into the system, even if the arguments for doing so in principle are quite strong.

Health-care professionals who make decisions about priorities are influenced in ways that lay them open to the accusation of being 'subjective'. One potential solution lies in allowing market mechanisms to make the decisions, since adherents to market principles advocate that the market provides a mechanism for a more efficient distribution of resources.

2.6   Rationing by markets

2.6.1   The notion of efficiency

The purpose of the market reforms was to make the health-care system more efficient, but efficiency itself is an ambiguous concept. To some people it simply means saving money (being economical), but this is not the meaning given to the term by economists, for whom a consideration of both costs *and benefits* is required. Normally, 'efficiency' is taken to mean 'value for money', where value refers to benefits and money refers to costs. But this does not match the economists' definition either, because money (i.e. financial outlay) is not necessarily a good indicator of the resources that have to be committed to get the benefits in question.

● What other costs need to be included in a definition of efficiency in health care?

■ In health care, the system does not meet any of the costs borne by patients and their families, and especially it does not meet the costs of their time.

However, even when we have sorted out which costs are included we are only half way to a definition of efficiency. At its lowest level the term might refer to finding ways to conduct a particular activity such as a surgical operation, or a day of hospital care, or a home visit by a GP, at a lower overall cost. In economics, this is called **technical efficiency**. However, even if every activity were conducted in a technically efficient manner, this would be no guarantee that the system as a whole is efficient, because it might be doing the wrong activities, for example offering surgical operations when treatment by drugs would be more efficient. This concept of higher-level efficiency is called **allocative efficiency**, and it poses a more fundamental question about whether any particular activity is worth doing at all, even when it is being done at the lowest possible cost!

Allocative efficiency requires us to compare costs with benefits, and benefits must be related to the system's objectives, which in the case of the NHS are to improve the health of the whole population as much as possible, and to reduce inequalities in health. This means that for the system to be truly efficient, each activity must contribute positively to these objectives to an extent that is justifiable given its true costs.

An historical example of an unnecessary procedure is tonsillectomy. There has been a dramatic reduction in the number of such operations performed over the past 30 years and many studies show that doctors have failed to agree about the need for surgery. At least since the 1970s, many tonsillectomy procedures are now thought to be unnecessary for the majority of children who present with recurrent tonsillitis.

Transferring costs to save money

The other problem is that people often save money by transferring costs to somebody else's budget, thereby claiming to have improved efficiency. This is obviously a false claim too, which is why economists insist that all resource costs must be counted, no matter who pays for them, and even if no-one pays for them! Somebody will always have made a sacrifice of some kind, and in principle it is the total value of those sacrificed alternatives that we need to measure to come to a sensible notion of cost. This returns us to the central dilemma of how we can balance the cost of one form of health care, such as a hip replacement, against the lost opportunity to devote resources to another, such as a home help, when both are equally desirable. This is another example of the problem of *opportunity cost* referred to earlier (Section 2.3.2).

Trials of efficacy?

In medicine, the theory and practice of the *clinical trial* have been developed specifically to answer the question, 'which health improvements does this intervention bring about for which kinds of patient?'[2] Unfortunately, such trials of efficacy have typically not been designed to answer the related question, 'and at what cost?'. The implication is that only the best is good enough, and costs (i.e. sacrifices) do not matter, which is a dangerous and unhelpful approach.

To respond more appropriately to the resource constraints faced by the NHS, there is increasing pressure to widen the scope of clinical trials and transform them into cost-effectiveness studies. But even when this happens it is commonly the case that only financial costs to the NHS are taken into account, so that they do not really address the fundamental efficiency issue adequately (Williams, 1997a).

[2] Clinical trials, particularly those where patients are randomly allocated to experimental or control groups (RCTs), are described in *Studying Health and Disease* (Open University Press, 2nd edn 1994; colour-enhanced 2nd edn 2001), Chapter 8.

2.6.2 The notion of equity

Clinical trials, and cost-effectiveness studies of clinical interventions, so far have only addressed efficiency issues concerned with the objective of improving people's health as much as possible. An important objective of the NHS has always been to reduce inequalities in health, and especially those related to people's socio-economic status. To address this equity issue requires clarity about what it is we are trying to make more equal. Policy of the late 1990s concentrated on making the distribution of resources more equal geographically, on guaranteeing equal access and on monitoring utilisation rates to see whether any particular 'at risk' group is failing to make proper use of the services that are provided. Hence the concern about take-up rates when screening, immunisation and health-promotion activities are provided, and the concern about late presentation of vulnerable people with potentially treatable conditions.

● Do activities such as screening inevitably reduce inequalities?

■ Such activities may actually widen the existing inequalities in health, if they are taken up and used more by those whose overall health prospects are good than by those whose overall health prospects are poor.

Thus, anti-smoking policies have been much more successful with people in professional and managerial occupations than with people in households where the principal wage-earner is an unskilled manual worker. It is already known that smoking is more prevalent in lower socio-economic groups and the data show that the differences are larger among younger than older people in most European countries (Cavelaars, 2000).

There are many different equity principles that can be brought to bear in this field, but the one that is most frequently appealed to is 'fairness'. This has two elements:

1 **Horizontal equity**, or treating equals equally, which requires specification of the respects in which people are to be held equal; this is usually achieved by specifying the converse, namely that people are *not* to be treated *unequally* because of age, gender, ethnicity, religion or sexual orientation.

2 **Vertical equity**, or treating unequals unequally according to their relative situation, which requires specification of the particular inequalities that are held to be unfair, and what sort of unequal treatment this justifies. Examples of vertical equity would include positive discrimination, on the basis of low social class or educational attainment.

● What principle of equity does postcode rationing offend?

■ It falls within the category of horizontal equity, because it is held that you should be treated equally no matter where you live.

2.6.3 Managing the problem of inequality

There is a moral dilemma here which is not widely recognised, and it is that, if we are going to reduce inequalities in people's lifetime experience of health, this means (amongst other things) making age at death less unequal between the different socio-economic groups. Looked at in a positive light, this means devoting relatively more resources to preventing premature deaths, i.e. deaths under the age of 60. In other words discriminating in favour of the young, as discussed in Case B (Box 2.1).

The other side of the same coin is that this means devoting relatively less resource to extending the length of life of those over the age of 60. In other words, discriminating against the old and all in the interests of fairness when seen as vertical equity! Many people, however, think that fairness when seen as horizontal equity requires no discrimination on grounds of age any more than on grounds of ethnicity or religion, so there is a clash of equity principles here. If you won't discriminate against older people, you may not reduce inequalities in lifetime experience of health; just as one might observe that if you won't discriminate against the rich, you cannot reduce inequalities in income. So equity does not always point in one direction.

2.6.4 The trade-off solution: equity or efficiency?

A difficult dilemma for policy analysis in health care arises if it turns out that it is more costly to bring about health improvements for the worse-off than it is to bring about similar health improvements for the better-off. This would bring the two principal objectives of equity and efficiency into conflict with each other. In order to reduce inequalities in health, it might be necessary to settle for a lower overall level of population health than would be feasible if we ignored the inequality issue. In the inelegant jargon of economics, this is referred to as the **equity–efficiency trade-off**, meaning that we have to decide how much *extra* weight to give to providing benefits for the worse-off compared with providing the same benefit for the better-off. That issue plays no role in clinical trials or in cost-effectiveness studies, where a given benefit is counted equally no matter who gets it. And it is difficult to see how it could be incorporated into such studies since ideas about the appropriate equity–efficiency trade-off may vary from context to context, and the results of such trials and studies tend to be used in a wide variety of contexts. It does imply that each purchasing authority should have a policy of its own about what weight it is going to give to the equity issue compared with the efficiency issue, and it should ensure that this policy is implemented consistently across all of the activities that it purchases.

2.7 Mechanisms to inform 'rational' rationing

2.7.1 Quality-of-life measurements

At whatever level the budget for the NHS is set, those who manage its budgets will have to think about its priorities. In order to improve the health of the population as much as possible, the NHS will have to compare the health gains from each activity with the costs of that activity, and concentrate resources where the marginal gain per pound's-worth of resources is greatest. It is necessary, therefore, to find some way of measuring health gains in a sufficiently general and versatile way that the health gains from quite dissimilar activities can be compared with each other. The commonest way of doing this in the past has been to measure survival rates, or life-years gained.

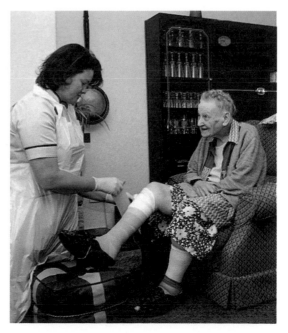

One of the most frequent tasks that community nurses perform is that of dressing leg ulcers of older people in the community. This routine type of care makes a significant contribution to people's quality of life. (Photo: Mike Levers)

● What is the problem with this measurement of health gain?

■ The measurement implies that only survival matters. However, people also care about the relief of pain and disability; many health-care activities have very little effect on life expectancy but are nevertheless extremely beneficial in relieving both pain and disability, for example hip replacements.

One way to compare inequalities in people's lifetime experience of health is to consider people's quality-adjusted life expectancy.

2.7.2 Quality-adjusted life expectancy

Measures of quality of life have been in existence since at least the 1970s. As a measure of healthiness and health gain, the **quality-adjusted life-year** (**QALY**) is one of the longest established. It combines years of life lost from premature death with a measure of quality-of-life after a particular treatment. It is not specific to any particular treatment or condition, and yet reflects the main attributes of health that ordinary people value most.[3] It therefore has the added advantage of not relying on professional judgements about what people value, but incorporates the values of the community that the NHS serves (i.e. the whole British public, in their various roles as patients, potential patients, citizens and taxpayers). Thus, one response to priority setting in relation to the objective of the NHS to maximise health gains has been to create 'cost-per-QALY league tables', and give priority to those activities which can deliver QALYs (i.e. health gains as valued by the general public) at the lowest cost (remembering that 'costs' include the sacrifices imposed on others by denying them the resources concerned).

2.7.3 QALYs and cost-per-QALY league tables

No-one would disagree that there is more to being healthy than living a long time, and that the quality of a person's life also counts for a lot. Living a long time with permanent disabilities and in continuous pain is not as good as living a long time in full health. There is a great deal of disagreement though about how best to weigh these different attributes of health one against another, when, for instance, the relief of pain requires the use of drugs which may shorten someone's life, or when, in order to relieve some disability, surgery is required which some people will not survive.

Some assert that these different elements are incommensurable, and in any case how can we weigh the risk of that great unknown, death, against living states with which we are at least familiar, such as severe disability? Others observe that, however difficult it may be, people make such judgements when deciding whether or not to accept some recommended treatment. Economists have formalised these processes in order to elicit the relative value that people attach to various states of *ill-health*.

Time trade-off (TTO) mimics the drug example above, and asks people how much of their life expectancy would they be prepared to sacrifice in order to get out of a specified (bad) health state and be healthy instead. The more time they are willing

---

[3] An alternative measure, the DALY or disability-adjusted life-year, is used by the World Health Organisation in international comparisons of disease burden; it combines years of life lost from premature death with a measure of loss of healthy life through disability. Different weights are attached to different disabilities in these calculations, which are discussed further in *World Health and Disease* (Open University Press, 3rd edn 2001), Chapter 3.

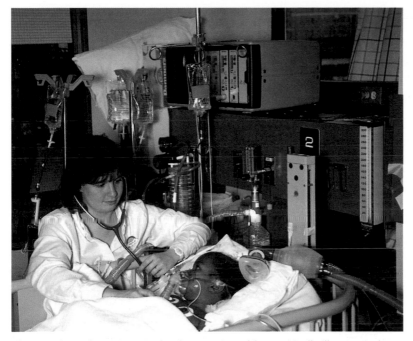

The experience for many people who are rescued from critically ill states is that life at whatever 'price' is worth hanging onto. This young person is receiving intensive life-saving care even though the outcome in terms of her quality of life is unknown. But under what circumstances might the sacrifices imposed on others be regarded as too great? (Photo: Science Photo Library)

to sacrifice, the worse that state must be. **Standard gamble** (SG) mimics the surgery example above, and asks people what risk of peri-operative death would they accept to get out of a specified (bad) health state and be healthy instead. The bigger the risk they would accept, the worse that state must be.

The values so elicited are expressed on a scale in which the value of being dead is rated at zero, and the value of full health is rated at 1.0. These values can be used as quality adjustments to produce the quality-adjusted life-year as a measure of healthiness and of health gains. Thus, if a health state is rated at 0.5, then two years in such a state would be regarded as equivalent to one year in full health, both being measured as 1 QALY. It can thus be used as a unit for comparing the effectiveness of different treatments for different conditions, where the benefits are different combinations of extra life-years, less pain and less disability.

To these data on the effectiveness of various treatments when given to different sorts of patient, we have to add data on the costs of those treatments. The resulting cost-effectiveness ratios for rival claimants on scarce resources make it possible to rank them in order of desirability according to how much it costs in each case to produce one QALY. Such rankings have been called 'Cost-per-QALY League Tables', and the first-ever British tables were published as long ago as 1985 (Williams, 1996). They included items which are represented in Table 2.1 (overleaf).

CABG is 'coronary artery bypass grafting', and is discussed further in Chapter 8. The purpose of this particular set of league tables was to work out how far to go in offering this treatment to patients with differing degrees of severity of coronary artery disease. 2VD means 'double vessel disease' which is a moderately severe presentation of coronary artery disease. LMD means 'left main disease', and when

Table 2.1 Summary of the costs and benefits of some selected treatments (in 1985).

Treatment	Extra costs (£000)	QALYs gained	Cost per QALY gained
haemodialysis in hospital	70	5	14
heart transplantation	23	4.5	5
CABG for moderate angina and 2VD	3	0.75	4
kidney transplantation	15	5	3
CABG for severe angina and LMD	2.85	2.75	1
hip replacement	3	4	0.75
pacemaker for heart block	3.5	5	0.7

Source: Williams, A. (1997) The Economics of Coronary Artery Bypass Grafting, in Culyer, A. J. and Maynard, A. K. (eds) *Being Reasonable about the Economics of Health*, pp. 238–48, Edward Elgar, Cheltenham.

it is the left main descending artery that is affected, this is the most severe presentation of the disease. You can see from Table 2.1 that it is more cost-effective to treat the more severe case than the less severe case, because the improvement in health is so much greater.

In a more fully articulated league table, which would include all of the options under review at the time, priority-setting would proceed by first purchasing those interventions which produce QALYs at the lowest costs, and working through the list item by item until the money runs out. This ensures that the greatest possible health gains are achieved with the resources available. If distributional issues are also important (i.e. if 'equity' in the distribution of health outcomes is important as well as 'efficiency' in maximising health outcomes), then the health gains (still in QALY terms) would have to be weighted differentially according to who is getting them. In all such league tables that have been published hitherto, QALYs have been regarded as of equal value no matter who gets them; an assumption for which there is also a strong ethical argument (Williams, 1996).

QALYs provide one example of a rationing mechanism, but there are other so-called 'neutral bodies' which serve to provide information to help decision-making on rationing, to which we now turn.

2.7.4 Health Technology Assessment

There are a number of relatively new sources of information about the cost-effectiveness of treatments. Many countries now have health technology agencies. In England and Wales, the **Health Technology Assessment (HTA) Programme** (NHS Executive, 1999), an advisory panel for the NHS, has several key functions, which are:

- to identify what knowledge gaps there are in the clinical and cost-effectiveness of health interventions;
- to prioritise and commission research to fill those gaps;
- to monitor the progress of these projects; and finally
- to disseminate information about the HTA programme.

The programme is a national one funded by the Department of Health (the equivalent agency in Scotland is the Health Technology Board for Scotland).

The **Centre for Reviews and Dissemination** (CRD) was established in 1994 to provide information on the effectiveness of treatments and the delivery and organisation of health care. CRD is part of the Cochrane Collaboration, an international network which prepares, maintains and disseminates reviews on the effects of health care.[4] Such mechanisms for rationing health care all aspire to provide information to help make rationing decisions more objective. The requirement to use this information is enshrined in NHS policy directives, such as the waiting list initiatives discussed in Section 2.3.1, but health-care decisions remain the responsibility of key decision-makers, particularly doctors.

2.7.5 NICE and other quality-improvement initiatives

The **National Institute for Clinical Excellence** (NICE) forms one part of the solution to remedy the current inequalities in health care. It was set up as a Special Health Authority for England and Wales in 1999 and is part of the NHS. The role of NICE is to provide clear national standards of what patients can expect from the NHS. To further this aim, NICE helps to promote clinical effectiveness (efficacy) through guidance to support frontline staff in the NHS. It does this by providing what it calls 'authoritative, robust and reliable guidance' on current 'best practice'. The guidance, often based on HTA reports, covers both individual health technologies, including medicines and medical devices, and diagnostic techniques and procedures and the clinical management of specific conditions.

Despite all these mechanisms, the question remains of whether or not the need for rationing simply derives from a lack of funds, and cannot be remedied by generating more information or redesigning organisations.

2.8 Is rationing due to underfunding?

The NHS currently (2001) has more resources available per head of population than ever before, but in 2000 the UK was still ranked 15th in spending per head on health care in countries of the Organisation for Economic Cooperation and Development (OECD) (World Health Organisation Report, 2000). There is an expectation that demand will increase, but how might demand decrease?

Frankel and colleagues (2000) argue that although the NHS is facing severe problems in meeting demand in some areas, a small increase in its resources would satisfy 'legitimate demands'. They use this term to mean demands generated by applying the conventional clinical indicators for treatment, as currently used by practitioners to decide whether a particular treatment should be offered to a particular patient. They also believe that the pressure on demand generated by an ageing population, by expensive new technologies, and by changing public expectations, are all greatly exaggerated. Furthermore, these 'pressures' may even work in the opposite direction if older people are getting healthier, if new technologies are cost-saving and if people are increasingly sceptical about the claimed efficacy of many treatments and so demand less health care. Although difficult choices have to be made about the use of scarce resources at a national level, these same pressures may or may not apply at a local level.

---

[4] The Cochrane Collaboration publishes an electronic database, the Cochrane Library, which consists mainly of systematic reviews of clinical trials. A subscription must be paid to access the full texts, but abstracts can be viewed free at (http://www.cochrane.org).

The health economist Bill New (2000) contests this view and observes that satisfying legitimate demand does not mean that there are no demands left unmet, and he points out that deciding what is and what is not a legitimate demand is in fact a rationing procedure. Moreover, if rationing is required at a national level, it is difficult to see how it can be avoided at the local level, since it is there that the difficult choices between patients will have to be made.

New believes that the future of the NHS will be more firmly assured by facing up to rationing issues and discussing them publicly in the hope that people's confidence in the NHS will thereby be strengthened. However, this aim leads to other dilemmas of how to select the best forum and people to make these decisions and what status to attribute to evidence in order to set priorities, when, at each stage of this process, there are competing interests and political pressures to evaluate or resist.

The resolution will depend first on the best balance to establish between the resources people are left to use according to their own wishes, and the resources allocated to provide public services for them according to some collective decisions. This balance focuses attention upon the appropriate level of taxation, since the NHS is essentially a tax-financed system, along with the social security system, education, defence and roads etc. It is between these rival claimants on taxpayers' money that the second level of policy making occurs, and here it is pertinent to remember that expenditures other than those on the NHS may make a major contribution to people's health, for example the relief of poverty, improved housing, a safer environment, better education, reduced unemployment, and so on. As noted earlier (Section 2.4), it is misleading to equate the budget for the NHS with the health budget, because the main determinants of health are not health-care activities at all but the material circumstances of people's lives (a subject that we return to in Chapter 9).

2.9   The role of economics in health care

Economics has been characterised as 'the dismal science', and on the face of it health economics, dealing as it does with the only two certainties in life (death and taxes), must be at the most dismal extreme of the dismal science. But taxes don't have to be higher than they need be, simply because those spending the taxpayers' money do so wastefully. And although death is unavoidable, it is often postponable, and until it comes, people's pain and disability can be reduced by the wise use of our limited resources. This requires all health-care professionals to take to heart the statement by the British Medical Association's Ethics Committee in 1999 that:

> Health professionals have an ethical duty to make the best use of the available resources and this means that hard decisions must be made. (BMA, 1999, p. 20)

Some of those hard decisions have just been sketched out, and we shall undoubtedly be hearing more and more of them as the priority-setting which has long been pursued implicitly and privately by doctors becomes increasingly explicit and publicly accountable. It will be a painful process for all concerned, and one that will test the maturity of the electorate and of the media. It will also test the capacity of a democratic system to face these inescapable dilemmas openly. Once Pandora's box has been opened, it cannot easily be closed again!

OBJECTIVES FOR CHAPTER 2

When you have studied this chapter, you should be able to:

2.1 Define and use, or recognise definitions and applications of, each of the terms printed in **bold** in the text.

2.2 Explain the extent to which health-care delivery is similar to or different from the process operating in other 'markets', including the relevance of the terms 'efficiency', 'cost-effectiveness' and 'equity' to the delivery of health care.

2.3 Outline some of the main ways in which the rationing of health care takes place and the ways in which decisions are taken about rationing.

QUESTIONS FOR CHAPTER 2

1 (*Objectives 2.1 and 2.2*)

Rosie Brown is a 60-year-old woman with symptoms of weight loss and anaemia for the past three months. Her GP referred her to a gastro-intestinal consultant at the general hospital. Rosie spent an anxious two months waiting for her appointment. On arrival at the out-patients department, Rosie and a friend who had accompanied her, were directed along a series of corridors to a waiting area, where they sat on chairs in a corridor facing the consultant's room.

Rosie saw the consultant for ten minutes, which included a physical examination. She felt upset that she was invited to answer specific questions but not given the opportunity to say what she wanted to, or to raise the many concerns she had. She was put onto another waiting list for a barium enema.

What information do you need to decide if this is an efficient use of NHS resources? What costs does this example raise?

2 (*Objectives 2.2 and 2.3*)

Following a serious road accident, Ben, a 45-year-old man, is admitted to the intensive therapy unit of St. Elsewhere Hospital, where he receives artificial ventilation and supportive therapy. His condition is thought to be very serious and his prognosis is poor but he remains stable for the next few days. Three days later, Hannah, a patient undergoing routine elective surgery, collapses and needs an ITU bed. With some ventilator support, Hannah's prognosis is thought to be good. However, the unit is full and Hannah has to be transferred 56 miles to the nearest available ITU bed.

What dilemmas does this example raise and to what extent might efficiency mechanisms resolve them in a way that is equitable?

3 (*Objective 2.3*)

How do measures of efficiency redress inequalities and meet the objective of providing health care in an equitable way?

CHAPTER 3

Dilemmas in health-care management

Study notes for OU students

Many of the dilemmas presented in this chapter arise from the successive reorganisations of the NHS in the 1990s, which were discussed in detail in *Caring for Health: History and Diversity* (Open University Press, 3rd edn 2001), Chapter 7. In particular, you will need to recall the general features of the 'internal market' in health care of the early 1990s, which established a division between purchasers and providers and created NHS Trusts and GP-fundholders; and also the reforms set in train since 1997, which are intended to create a 'seamless service' at local level, with GPs taking the lead in locality commissioning of services to meet local needs. It would be useful to look again at Figure 7.5 in that book, to remind yourself of the 'command structure' of the NHS, from the Secretary of State for Health down to local managers and providers. We also assume that you recall the general features of the main debates about the management of nursing, which were discussed in Chapters 6 and 7 of *Caring for Health: History and Diversity*.

In Section 3.6 of the present chapter, you will be referred to an article by Chris Ham, entitled 'Improving NHS performance: human behaviour and health policy', which can be found in *Health and Disease: A Reader* (Open University Press, 3rd edn 2001). This chapter was written by David Cox who is a Professor and Associate Dean Academic, Faculty of Health and Community Care at the University of Central England.

3.1 Introduction

Very high hopes have been placed on the idea that managerial actions and techniques can produce an efficient and effective health service that meets public expectations. But what does this mean in practice? This chapter considers the quest for an appropriate NHS management structure in more detail. In particular, at a national level, how does the government manage the NHS and, at a more local and operational level, what do managers do when they manage? This chapter will cover these issues from the perspective of government, hospital managers and professional health-care staff. It highlights:

- the dilemmas of management and the range of managerial control strategies that might be relevant to health-care organisations;
- the dilemmas for British governments in seeking to implement their policies through management strategies;
- the dilemmas facing local service managers and middle managers in NHS Trusts;
- the dilemmas created for professionals by their changing relationships with management;
- the management dilemmas in primary care as general practitioners (GPs) become both purchasers and providers of health-care services.

We begin with an example of what appears to be an insignificant issue but one that has raised much public concern.

3.1.1 Why is hospital cleaning still a problem?

In the summer of 2000, the Labour government produced a substantial plan which indicated the future direction of NHS development and investment in England (Department of Health, 2000a). Arrangements for the other countries of the UK differ in certain respects, but the issues remain much the same. Public consultations leading to *The NHS Plan* revealed widespread dissatisfaction with standards of hospital cleanliness and a demand for the return of the 'matron' who, as part of her overall responsibility for hospital-patient care, would oversee cleaning standards. The first appointment of the new matrons — each responsible for a small number of wards — was announced in spring 2001. After many years of trying to manage cleaning through the strategy of compulsory competitive tendering, the proposal was for a return to traditional management in the form of a nurse manager directly giving orders.

It is paradoxical that at the start of the 21st century there was still a basic managerial problem about ensuring that hospital wards were adequately cleaned. Lord Hunt, a Health Minister at the time, placed hospital cleanliness high on the list of priorities for achieving comfort, convenience and dignity for hospital patients. In July 2000 he declared that: '… each Trust would draw up action plans to set work priorities and that by the autumn all Trusts will have been inspected by Patient Environment Action Teams. These teams, which will include representatives of the Patients' Association and NHS professionals such as infection control nurses, will help make sure that action plans are implemented so that patients start to see positive changes.' He also claimed that 'a good quality environment is essential to give a feeling of well being and confidence in the NHS. Patients have a right to receive treatment, and recover, in clean and comfortable surroundings. The NHS Hospital Clean-up initiative will help ensure that all Trusts meet acceptable standards of cleanliness for the benefit of patients and NHS staff.' (Hunt, 2000).

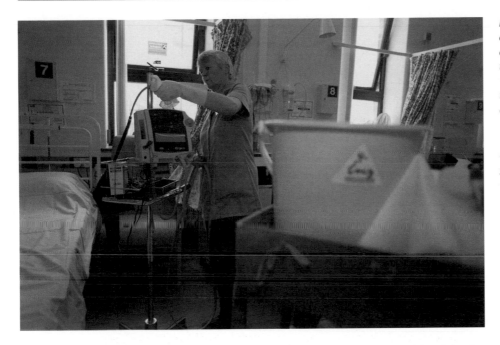

Many UK hospitals are old buildings which are difficult to maintain, but they remain the public 'face' of the NHS and their cleanliness continues to represent 'standards of care'. Therefore, a clean hospital translates into good quality care. (Photo: United National Photographers)

The rest of this chapter explores the roots of the 'management problem' in the NHS.

3.1.2 Management and the problem of control

The most fundamental question for management in large organisations is how to direct the work of other people while controlling costs. It is a difficult and challenging task. If it is hard to ensure basic cleaning, then trying to control standards of health care, complex medical procedures, spending patterns, employment policies, customer care or waiting lists is much more challenging. At a national level, UK governments can be held accountable for what happens or does not happen in the NHS anywhere in the country, at any time of day or night. Cancelled operations, 'trolley waits', medical mistakes, hospital closures, health authority overspends, ambulance response times and patient aggression or self-harm are examples of incidents that can end up with the Secretary of State for Health. A former Secretary of State for Health, Virginia Bottomley, captured the extent of responsibility attached to this role:

> I ... regarded myself as really like an executive chairman. I felt enormously responsible and 24 hours a day concerned about the NHS. (quoted in Ham, 2000, p. 42)

As Robert Baggott, a Reader in Public Policy (at De Montfort University), claimed:

> ... responsibility for the NHS is rather like throwing away a boomerang. When things go seriously wrong, ministers have great difficulty in distancing themselves from the problems of the service (Baggott, 1998, p. 159).

It is this pressure of accountability that has driven the quest for new management arrangements which stretch down from the Department of Health to hospital and primary-care managers, and to the professionals and other staff who work with them delivering health care at a local level.

3.2 The dilemmas of management: delegation and control

A manager is accountable for the work of other people, and all managers are faced with the problem of delegation. The dilemma is that too little delegation stifles initiative, overloads the 'centre' and creates inefficiency; whereas too much delegation might mean that managers are blamed for errors, mistakes and cost overruns. To resolve this dilemma, managers search for an optimum balance between control and delegation. Government ministers and managers at the centre of the NHS are forced to delegate tasks for which they are accountable, and therefore need to develop strategies and techniques to control effectively their staff at the front line.

● Suggest where the delegation would begin in the NHS and which front-line staff or organisations might carry out the delegated work.

■ In the NHS, government is the central locus of control, delegating work to regional and local health authorities, Trust boards and local managers.[1]

Here, hospital kitchen staff are working in an assembly line – serving patients' meals. Dividing health-care work into 'tasks' has received criticism on the basis that it reduces 'caring' into mechanical activities, and erodes job satisfaction. (Photo: Mike Levers)

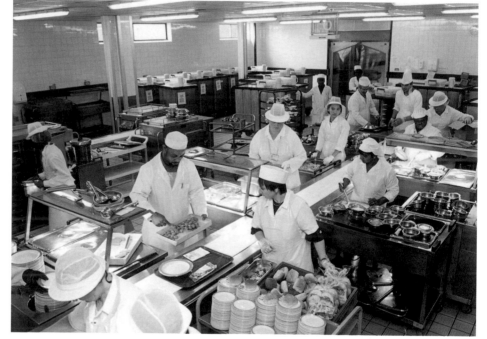

The problem of control over delegated tasks occurs at all levels. A first-line supervisor may be able to issue clear instructions and observe tasks being done. A nurse ward-manager relies on the professional training and socialisation of her or his staff but reinforces this with instructions, handovers and clinical supervision. General managers divide an organisation's tasks and priorities into departments and roles, employ specialists, issue job descriptions, rules, budgets and occasionally orders. They then devise a variety of 'reporting' mechanisms to monitor conformity with policies and guidance, assess variances and check standards in the services for which they are accountable. Work that requires initiative, creativity and commitment is harder to manage, particularly if specialist expertise is involved.

[1] The relationships between these sectors in England is discussed in detail in *Caring for Health: History and Diversity* (Open University Press, 3rd edn 2001), Chapter 7; see Figure 7.5.

As organisations grow, new monitoring mechanisms are introduced such as periodic reviews, information systems, inspections and audits, which together constitute **performance management**. A key aspect of this process is the issuing (or agreeing) of targets and performance indicators, which can be carefully monitored. In the modern NHS therefore, we find a repertoire of strategies to control this large organisation. Practice and theory provide strategies that can be used in varied and changing mixes, as illustrated in Box 3.1.

> **Box 3.1   Management strategies for control in the health service**
>
> - Division of labour or specialisation — dividing the work up into manageable units and roles (Trusts, directorates, wards, teams, job specifications). In health care, professionalisation is very important, highly trained specialists have unique skills and their training and socialisation aim to ensure trustworthy and reliable performance.
>
> - Hierarchy or centralisation — introducing various levels of supervisory or management roles to co-ordinate and control 'subordinates' (ward managers, general managers, chief executives).
>
> - Rules or standardisation — prescribing how tasks should be carried out (guidelines, procedures, standard financial instructions, policies, including National Service Frameworks).
>
> - Records or formalisation — maintaining evidence that rules have been followed, monies and activities accounted for (standard data sets, financial returns, medical and nursing notes, computerised information systems, etc.).
>
> - Management by contract is an alternative to hierarchy — contract specifications, market testing and the purchasing of services or components, linking payments to performance (competitive tendering of ancillary services, the 'internal market' of the NHS 1991–7).
>
> - Management culture and style — attempts to change the way managers and staff carry out their work and improve their motivation (changing language and self image, use of terms like entrepreneurship, mission statement, dynamic, pro-active, leadership, partnership).

Managing an organisation of the size and complexity of the NHS stretches managerial strategies to the limit. Many of the changes in the management of the NHS since 1990 have been influenced by management trends from the private sector. The industrialist Sir Adrian Cadbury spoke about these changes in management culture:

> We will want, in future, to break these organisations down into their separate business units and to give those units freedom to compete in their particular markets. Large companies will become more like federations of small enterprises — not because 'small is beautiful' but because big is expensive and inflexible. I would expect tomorrow's companies to concentrate on the core activities of their business, relying for everything else on specialised suppliers who would compete for their custom. (Cadbury, quoted in Klein, 1995, p. 139)

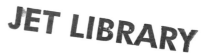

● What does the language tell you about the change of emphasis in culture?

■ The language includes an emphasis on outputs, performance measures and competition between small units.

This managerial strategy from the private sector influenced the introduction of NHS Trusts and the internal market in 1991. In any large organisation, the process of coordination and control produces tensions between the top levels (or centre) and the front line (or periphery), where services are delivered and subject to the complexity of everyday reality and pressures. Each management strategy produces its own limitations and costs. It is a common characteristic that in an organisation like a hospital, employees establish their own group loyalties, pride, commitments and local knowledge. It is inevitable that changing the structure in pursuit of the next reorganisation will provoke resistance. Consequently, protecting the organisation from top-down directives is a common concern of managers at the front line. A market approach can cut the costs of running a large bureaucratic organisation, but also carries new transaction costs associated with running an internal market. These include the managerial tasks of tendering, designing specifications and marketing services.

● What are the distinctive features of health-care staff that make the NHS different from other types of organisation?

■ Health-care organisations employ many medical and other professionals whose skills and expertise are critical to their core tasks and on whom the lives of patients depend. Clinical decisions are central to health care and the ability to make these decisions is dependent upon expert knowledge.

Management decisions that threaten to undermine professional expertise can escalate into highly emotive territorial disputes. Conversely, expert decisions can undermine management in ways that managers cannot control — or sufficiently understand to question them. Anslem Strauss and colleagues observed that in health care there was a 'negotiated order' formed from loose coalitions of professionals, whose activities and relationships had to be negotiated and facilitated in order to ensure patient care (Strauss *et al.*, 1963). Although medical power predominated, other professions and occupations also maintained their own subordinate domains of autonomous activity. Therefore, rather than controlling the work of professionals, the health-service administrator served as coordinator and provider of facilities in which the professionals could work.

This negotiated order, built around carefully constructed divisions of labour, has been challenged since the 1980s by the strategies of general management, resource management techniques and 'customer care'.

3.3 Dilemmas for governments: determined to devolve, condemned to intervene

3.3.1 Hands-on management from the top

Managerial direction down the chain of command and control from government comes in two forms:

● driving major policy change; and

● monitoring the day-to-day performance of the NHS.

Where there is the determination to achieve change and see the existing service reconfigured to the shape required by the latest 'reforms', the managerial drive will be strong, even when the outcome is purported to be a more diverse and locally managed service.

The result is that UK Secretaries of State for Health, and their junior health ministers, find themselves drawn into taking responsibility for day-to-day matters within the NHS, when in theory they should only be concerned with the broad strategic direction of the service.

3.3.2 Delegation versus accountability

In the early 1990s, when the process of delegation and devolution in the NHS began with the introduction of the internal market, the Conservative government used Trust autonomy, competition between health-care providers, and GP-fundholding to give the impression that central control had been relaxed and operational matters were a 'local responsibility'.

The Labour government's policies from 1997 were less of a challenge to established NHS norms, but the implementation strategy was concerned with forcing the pace and ensuring change. They faced similar dilemmas of achieving change through central control without appearing to stifle initiative and local and professional leadership within the service. In 1997, the White Paper *The New NHS Modern Dependable* (Department of Health, 1997) was to be implemented through very tight deadlines; guidance and circulars poured forth from Whitehall and dominated health-service managerial agendas. The language of business and competition was ruled out in a national 'caring' service and replaced by a rhetoric of partnership, a duty to enhance quality (as well as maintain financial control) and references to the NHS 'family'. This in itself was an attempt to recreate the 'unique culture' of the NHS and invoke its founding principles,[2] as well as open the way to 'modernisation'.

In the early years of their administration, the 1997 Labour government made much of maintaining national standards, in contrast to the variation in service quality — the postcode lottery — that may have been permitted by giving market forces a free rein.

● Why is increased central government control an inevitable consequence of the desire to 'universalise' the best standards?

■ Standard setting at the national level means that there must be monitoring of quality control locally against centrally determined targets.

An extension of the control strategies that guaranteed these standards included instructions, oversight, National Service Frameworks (which set standards and define services for particular service or care groups, put in place programmes to support implementation, and establish performance measures), performance management, new appointments and threats of managers being dismissed in the event of failure.

● What economic constraints make it difficult for UK governments to delegate the management of the NHS to health-service managers?

[2] The founding principles of the NHS in 1948 to be an inclusive service offering quality health care 'free at the point of delivery' are discussed in *Caring for Health: History and Diversity* (Open University Press, 3rd edn 2001), Chapters 5 and 6.

■ The NHS consumes large amounts of public money which is the focus of public and media interest. As a national service, there is pressure to ensure equity of provision through quality and expenditure across the country, yet the size, diversity and complexity of the service inevitably generates untoward variations which demand intervention from beyond local management.

3.3.3 Attempts to balance intervention and 'earned autonomy'

The dilemma of balancing the need for centralisation without stifling local creativity was recognised in *The NHS Plan* (Department of Health, 2000a), which claimed that local hospitals cannot be run from Whitehall. NHS staff had responded to the consultation before publication of the plan by expressing a wish for local autonomy and less central control. The government's response is encapsulated in the following extracts.

> Because we trust people on the front line, the centre will do only what it needs to do; then there will be maximum devolution to local doctors and other health professionals …. The centre will set standards, monitor performance, put in place a proper system of inspection, provide back up to assist modernisation of the service and, where necessary, correct failure. Intervention will be in inverse proportion to success: a system of earned autonomy. The centre will not try and take every last decision. There will be progressively less central control and progressively more devolution as standards improve and modernisation takes hold. (Department of Health, 2000a, para. 6.6, p. 57)

Through a **traffic light** system (see below), the plan promised to find a middle way between overcentralisation and fragmentation, allowing local innovation and leadership, within the Performance Assessment Framework (PAF), a framework of national standards and inspection to ensure quality control and equity. Further:

> Depending on their performance against the Performance Assessment Framework, all NHS organisations (Health Authorities, NHS Trusts, Primary Care Groups, Primary Care Trusts, and Health Action Zones) will for the first time annually and publicly be classified as 'green', 'yellow' or 'red'. Criteria will be set nationally but assessment will be by Regional Offices with independent verification by the Commission for Health Improvement. (*ibid*, para. 6.26, p. 63)

> Red organisations will be those who are failing to meet a number of the core national targets. Green organisations will be meeting all core national targets and will score in the top 25 per cent of organisations on the Performance Assessment Framework, taking account of 'value added'. Yellow organisations will be meeting all or most national core targets, but will not be up in the top 25 per cent of Performance Assessment Framework performance. So red status will result from poor absolute standards of performance, triggering action to ensure that a 'floor' level of acceptable performance is achieved throughout the NHS. Green status reflects both outstanding absolute performance against core national targets and relative performance against the wider Performance

Assessment Framework measures, serving as an incentive for continuous improvement on the part of all organisations. The 25 per cent threshold for green status will be reviewed periodically. (*ibid*, para. 6.27, p. 63)

3.4   Dilemmas for health-service managers

Thus far we have looked at the intrinsic dilemmas of management and the way in which UK governments have sought to manage the NHS. In this section, we ask who are the managers and how do they carry out their responsibilities within the NHS system?

3.4.1   Who are the managers in the NHS?

Figure 3.1 provides a summary of the numbers of staff employed by the NHS in England.

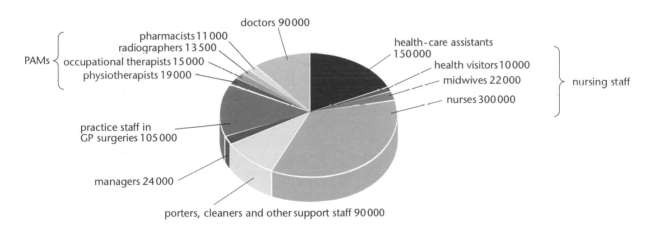

Figure 3.1   *Hospital and Community Health Services staff by main staff groups on a typical day in the NHS. (Source: Department of Health, 2000,* The NHS Plan: a plan for investment, a plan for reform, *Cmd 4818, The Stationery Office, London)*

The NHS Plan promises additional investment in the NHS, including 7 500 more consultants, 2 000 more GPs, 20 000 extra nurses and 6 500 extra therapists and 1 000 more medical school places (p. 11). No promises are made about extra managers although the promised 7 000 extra beds and over 100 new hospitals must generate some additional managerial work in ensuring implementation. Later in *The NHS Plan*, it is stated that 'on a typical day' there are 24 000 managers which accounts for 2.7 per cent of a workforce of 863 500 (*ibid*, p. 24).

The key source for NHS management job advertisements is the weekly *Health Service Journal*. A typical issue will have around 200 jobs advertised, spanning a range of managerial posts. These include:

- Chief Executive positions (in Health Authorities and Trusts). These senior posts are concerned with implementing policy, balancing the books of their organisations, and wrestling with issues of reorganisation and reconfiguration of services and organisations.
- Functional posts at various levels of seniority in the key support services of finance, human resources, estates and information technology (IT).

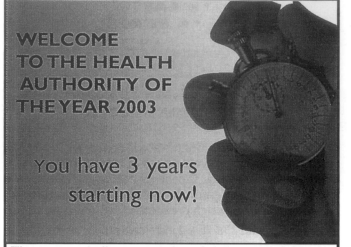

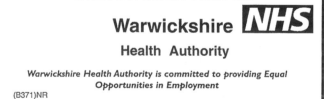

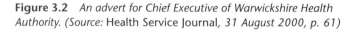

Figure 3.2 *An advert for Chief Executive of Warwickshire Health Authority. (Source: Health Service Journal, 31 August 2000, p. 61)*

- Middle management posts of two types. First, there are posts managing directorates or sections of a Trust, often as business managers working alongside a clinical director. Secondly, there are many project manager positions leading developments in particular fields, such as chronic heart-disease services, which involve leading teams from across a Trust or from several organisations.

If managerial culture is embodied in the use of language, then the wording of advertisements illuminates the current climate within which health-service managers are expected to fit. Figure 3.2 is a typical advertisement. Look at it carefully.

- Make a list of the key words in the advertisement and consider what the language tells us about the type of manager they were seeking.

- The advertisement uses words like 'challenge', 'inspirational leader', 'drive' and 'determination', together with 'integrity' and 'people skills' — all of which convey the managerial style and culture of competition that this Health Authority aspires to.

There is a competitive element in the ambition to become 'Health Authority of the Year' (an annual award like an Oscar from the *Health Service Journal*), while it is clear that the financial 'bottom line' and meeting 'national and local priorities' are critical. This leader will also need to be able to develop 'partnerships' with others and accept the awesome responsibility for the health of 503 000 people.

You might like to reconsider the factors that determine the health of populations[3] and consider how far one manager, however skilled and well paid, can really have much effect. Although the value of their role in comparison with that of front-line key NHS staff is contested, it would still seem that health workers in general are undervalued (as we discuss in Chapter 5).

[3] Socio-economic determinants of ill health in the UK are discussed in detail in *World Health and Disease* (Open University Press, 3rd edn 2001), Chapters 9 and 10.

3.4.2 Changing cultures

Many of the successive reorganisations of the NHS have explicitly called for 'cultural change' among NHS staff. **Culture** in this context means shared patterns of belief, meaning and behaviour and there has been much attention to this concept in recent management theory. In their study of the implementation of the Griffiths Report (Griffiths, 1983) into NHS management, Phil Strong and Jane Robinson (1988) show the inspirational momentum that characterised the introduction of *general management* and the morale and self-esteem of the new generation of district general managers. Thus:

> The (Griffiths) report captured the spirit of the age in a way managed by no other document. Many of those we observed, interviewed or heard lecture were deeply committed to the new way of doing things. In this heady atmosphere, a new organisational and moral vision was outlined. For this was both a new way of structuring the health service and a moral crusade. (Strong and Robinson, 1988, p. 54)

More recently, Christopher Pollitt, Johnston Birchall and Keith Putman (1998) showed that there was a similar process of cultural transition associated with the introduction of the internal market and Trust status in the early 1990s, and once again an intensive cycle of management conferences and seminars supported networking and the achievement of personal change. They argue:

> It was actually quite hard for senior NHS Trust managers to behave 'appropriately' during the early days of the provider market .... They were under fierce and contradictory pressures from the government. On the one hand they were supposed to behave dynamically and entrepreneurially, but, on the other, strong messages from the centre told them not to do things that might cause adverse media attention. (Pollitt *et al.*, 1998, p. 97)

As the internal market reforms slowly developed, however, the NHS accommodated incremental change. Trust status and market survival also helped legitimise the managerial role and consolidate the division of responsibilities between managers and doctors. Christopher Pollitt and colleagues stated that in a semi-competitive provider market, everyone in a Trust knew that they would sink or swim together, and there was both peer and managerial pressure on anyone obstructing progress, being inefficient or falling behind productivity norms (Pollitt *et al.*, 1998, p. 98).

3.4.3 The rhetoric of NHS management

People use language to rationalise and describe their lives and this rhetoric does not always correspond to reality. The transformations of the **'new public management'** (introduced in the late 1990s) included an emphasis on output and measures of performance, the introduction of competition and private-sector styles of management, seeing patients as consumers, and increasing audit and regulatory control over health professionals[4]. If these changes are to have any impact on patient care, the rhetoric must be reflected in reality in the different ways in which people working in the NHS make decisions, behave and carry out their roles.

---

[4] The new public management is discussed in greater detail in *Caring for Health: History and Diversity* (Open University Press, 3rd edn 2001), Chapter 7.

The rhetoric that managers employ to persuade, cajole and facilitate the processing of work in their organisations occupies a significant part of their role. Reacting to a rapid succession of issues is a world away from the idealised theories of planning, organising and controlling.

3.4.4 The power of key managers: the reality

In the study by Christopher Pollitt and colleagues (1998, see Section 3.4.2), they interviewed key managers in four NHS Trusts to explore the extent to which they were able to exercise the freedoms and powers in hospitals or units that wished to become independent of Health Authorities and become NHS Trusts. These powers enabled the acquisition and disposal of assets, borrowing, retention of surpluses and reserves, the setting up of their own management structures, and much greater freedom to employ staff, including medical staff and to determine conditions of service. However, the research showed that these alleged benefits were rarely mentioned by the Trust managers. Instead, as they claim:

> The most emphasised and most frequently cited motive (for applying for Trust status) was the more negative one of simply escaping from the control of the District Health Authority (DHA) and/or Regional Health Authority (RHA). (Pollitt *et al.*, 1998, p. 68)

The new Trusts faced significant financial constraints from the internal market, which produced some financial crises, major job losses (600 at Guy's Hospital in London) and rationalisations of older hospitals in major cities. The contracts between purchasers and providers sharpened-up managerial awareness of income and expenditure imbalances. This provoked radical restructuring in many Trusts to contain costs and prevent hospital activity exceeding the levels specified in their service contracts with purchasers locally.

3.4.5 The dilemma of overperformance

In an NHS Trust, a key management dilemma relates to the control of 'overperformance'. If only a certain number of procedures, for example hip replacements, were specified in the contract with a purchaser (usually the local health authority or GP-fundholding practice), and were therefore paid for, clinicians had to be restrained from admitting more patients (except from additional contracts) until a new annual contract began. Clearly, clinicians never admit patients who do not need surgical operations, so the limits on the number of procedures were being influenced by the contract and the purchasers' funds, rather than by need.

- What do you think was one of the key consequences of these limits on the health service?

- Delayed operations and increased waiting lists and times created public concern and controversy over a 'two-tier' service, in which patients were 'deferred' in localities where the contract had already been fulfilled.

This dilemma for both the government and NHS managers (not to mention frustrated clinicians forced to slow down and patients forced to wait) was to some extent resolved by directing extra funding to reduce waiting lists, and by three-year service and financial frameworks introduced to provide some flexibility (as discussed in Chapter 2).

Managers are surrounded by a rhetoric of performance, effectiveness and the achievement of targets. A problem for managers is to know how they will be judged and which *performance indicators* suggest that they and their Trust are doing a good job. For Christopher Pollitt and colleagues' (1998) respondents, rather than clinical effectiveness, the crucial measurements in 1994 and 1995 seemed to be finance and *The Patients' Charter*[5] measures (especially waiting times), together with **activity level** (the number of finished consultant episodes, day cases and so on) in each specialty.

3.4.6 Dilemmas facing middle managers

Managers in NHS Trusts are mainly concerned with the detailed implementation of corporate policy and ensuring the day-to-day smooth running of the units and departments in which they work, at the same time they have to act within the requirements of the government and the Trust. Both require them to perform a balancing act of interests which involves making choices between less than favourable options.

For example, Graeme Currie carried out an empirical qualitative study into the role of middle managers in the NHS (Currie, 1999a; 1999b). He points out that while middle management expanded in the 1980s and early 1990s, this position began to change.

Graeme Currie's study looked at the role middle managers play in implementing strategic policies and change. He showed that those he interviewed did more than merely implement policy changes and monitor NHS performance. They were an essential link between major corporate or Trust level policy and the day-to-day operations. They also interpreted and negotiated the implementation of policies in the local context. In practice, the managers resisted central policies that would not have worked in their area and initiated alternative approaches that

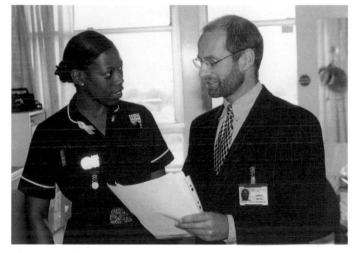

The image of NHS managers as 'men in grey suits' is a popular one and difficult to change, even though a substantial proportion are women. Here a hospital manager talks to a senior ward nurse. (Photo: Mike Levers)

were more appropriate. The study showed how they worked within broad strategic frameworks, which allowed them some discretion and influence on how the strategy emerged. Middle managers, through membership of working groups, also had some input into how corporate strategies evolved at the level of the Trust Board. Local and operational knowledge gave them some limited influence, provided that their actions were consistent with overall government requirements and the corporate view of the Trust.

Two factors were involved. First, there was a wider managerial trend towards *delayering* in which front-line health professionals were given more responsibility to manage their own work, and various supervisory layers were removed. Secondly, popular criticism of 'men in grey suits' managing the NHS was followed by successive government ministers who were determined to cut management costs and set tough targets to ensure savings.

[5] *The Patients' Charter* was introduced in England in 1991, and promoted information and choice to patients represented as individual consumers.

3.5 Managerial dilemmas for health professionals

3.5.1 Managing hospital doctors

Hospital doctors, and especially consultants, are a key group whose actions and decisions determine much about the quality and cost of a Trust's services. Admission into hospital, ordering of diagnostic tests, treatments and procedures, length of stay, and patient discharge into the community are the essential workflow of an acute hospital and they depend on clinical decisions most often made by doctors. A central problem for health-service managers is how to exercise control over doctors. After all, it is senior doctors who commit much of the organisation's resources, determine much of what happens to patients, and enjoy substantial **clinical autonomy**, i.e. the right to make choices based on clinical judgement.

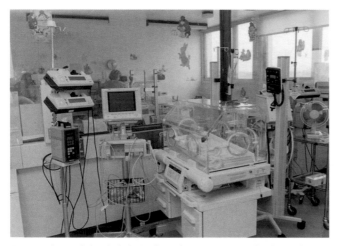

Doctors have defended their clinical autonomy in the face of managerial challenges, particularly (as discussed in Chapter 1) in centres of clinical excellence and showcases of modern medicine such as neonatal intensive-care units. (Photo: Mike Levers)

Doctors also belong to a strong collective organisation and senior doctors enjoy the financial independence that results from high salaries and ample alternative employment opportunities, including private practice. The dilemma for managers resides in the conflict between achieving targets without upsetting senior doctors. If managers just issue 'top-down' orders to consultants, they risk alienating a powerful vested interest and being held accountable for unanticipated consequences such as cancelled operations. However, without influencing consultants' behaviour, managers cannot achieve key objectives in terms of government priorities on cost control, clinical processes (such as audit) or waiting lists. Managers have tried to resolve this dilemma in several ways.

An important starting point has been a series of changes in the employment conditions of consultants. From a position where consultants' contracts were held at the regional level of the NHS and local hospital managers had no say in appointments, workloads or the important 'merit' payments, successive reforms have led to contracts being held by Trusts. By the end of the 1990s, Trusts were routinely making clinical appointments, and managers had an influence on 'merit' payments and agreeing work plans with consultants.

Doctors as managers

The main managerial response to the dilemma of managing doctors has been to co-opt senior doctors into specific medical management responsibilities and roles and especially to the key roles of directors. The creation of NHS Trusts from 1991 required that every Trust have a **medical director** who participates in full collective responsibility for the Trust's affairs. Specific duties include medical disciplinary matters, clinical risk management, medical staffing, research and development, clinical audit and medical training. These are demanding roles and medical directors are faced with the decision of whether to give up clinical work; most maintain clinical sessions out of interest, the need to retain credibility with colleagues and to give themselves an exit strategy after their term of office.

The main complaints from a survey of medical directors carried out by the British Association of Medical Managers included poor preparation for their managerial role, the lack of a career structure, inadequate financial rewards and lack of support. Despite this, 92 per cent said they would choose to repeat the experience if given the opportunity (*Health Service Journal*, editorial, 20 April 2000, p. 22).

Two medical directors who featured in the study reported in the *Health Service Journal* provide an insight into the experience of being a director. Michael Porte stated:

> The very term medical director is a misnomer — I direct virtually nothing. I have to influence, cajole, facilitate, persuade and co-ordinate. (*Health Service Journal*, 2000, p. 23)

Shirley Remington said:

> Today I have been at a meeting for resuscitation co-ordinators to discuss training, an appraisal meeting, a continuing medical education meeting for anaesthetics, and I am drafting a clinical perspective on the rising admission pressures and then have a management board meeting to attend. (*ibid*, p. 25)

Clinical directorates

While medical directors play a key role in managing medical matters at Trust level, the introduction of **clinical directorates** has been a more fundamental way of bringing the day-to-day work of consultants under a measure of managerial control. The work of an acute hospital is divided into specialist sub-groups each with its medical and nursing staff, Professions Allied to Medicine (PAMs), administrative support and allocated resource of beds, theatre time, pathology services and pharmaceuticals. (The role of PAMs is discussed further in Chapter 5.) These clinical directorates could then plan their work and became the basis for the difficult management process of systematically costing operations and treatments and making comparisons between hospitals and units.

Since the managerial changes of the 1990s, the clinical directorate has become an almost universal feature of acute hospitals. Clinical directorates enabled negotiations about the volume, costs and quality of treatments with purchasers to be devolved down to a clinical level. As hospital and Trust managers struggled with scarce resources, bed numbers were reduced, innovations like day surgery and keyhole surgery spread rapidly and clinical directorates were rationalised, often with consolidation of consultant teams from different hospitals into larger, more efficient groupings.

The issues of leadership and coordination for a clinical directorate became paramount, and the **clinical director** position emerged as a hybrid post in charge of each directorate but also engaged in clinical care. Clinical directors' appointments were often made from the elected representatives or nominees of groups of consultants and were different from medical directors in that they were responsible for specific clinical areas.

● Why would it be important that clinical directors were elected positions?

■ In order to be seen as legitimate managers, clinical directors needed to have credibility both with the other health professionals who are their colleagues and with the Trust management.

Juggling these twin responsibilities usually means that clinical directors keep a clinical workload and do the management work part-time. Directorate teams usually include a business manager, doing the day-to-day managerial work, a nursing manager and often a full or part-time accountant. A group of consultants without an effective clinical director would lose out in the competition for resources — beds, budgets and contracts. Where directorate teams failed to attract sufficient resources or maintain a critical mass of work and specialist cover, they could be threatened both by the purchasing decisions of Health Authorities and GP-fundholders, and more immediately by the relevant Royal College which could withdraw, or threaten to withdraw, postgraduate training status and with it the essential workforce of junior doctors and registrars. Trying to balance these demands with the day-to-day management of clinical care has proved to be a demanding role for the new corps of 'doctor-managers'.

The dilemma for clinical directors is that they are involved both in the struggle for finite resources and in trying to control members of their own directorate. As one clinical director commented, 'I often feel we are mainly ciphers. We are here mainly to control our consultant colleagues' (Pollitt et al., 1998, p. 98). However, this research showed how effective the encroachment of managerial controls has been. For example, 'breaking down waiting list and waiting time information by consultant, permitted senior managers and doctors to exert greater leverage against those who appeared to be out of line' (*ibid*, p. 98). Despite external pressure and competitive demands, there was a need to universalise effective health-care delivery.

3.5.2 Quality control

The mechanisms of quality control of medical performance have developed from confidential peer reviews and clinical audit in the early 1990s, to the more explicit and transparent quality-assurance techniques associated with **clinical governance**. This is defined as a framework through which NHS organisations are accountable for continuously improving the quality of their services and safeguarding high standards of care.

Clinical governance was a major element of the 1997 Labour government's NHS policy. It was a framework that combined national guidance and inspection with requirements on Trusts to take corporate responsibility for the quality and standards of clinical care. At Trust level, this included procedures for assessing risks, responding to complaints, auditing performance and ensuring the continual professional development and updating of all clinical staff.

From the 1980s, medical audit procedures were encouraged by the Department of Health with incentives and funding for administrative support. The Confidential Enquiries into Peri-operative Deaths (CEPOD) involved fellow doctors (peers) reviewing deaths during operations and ensuring that any lessons were learnt and conveyed to the surgical team concerned. These proceedings were confidential. They could not be used by management to exert control, and patients' relatives were similarly excluded for fear of litigation.

● On what grounds could it be argued that keeping the results of CEPOD enquiries confidential was, on balance, likely to benefit patients?

■ Surgeons are performing difficult tasks with patients whose chances of recovery could be very poor. Keeping information within the profession meant that procedures and skills could be improved through learning, but without the perverse incentive of consultants avoiding operating on patients where the risks of failure were high from fear of litigation.

Gradually, the mutual peer-review processes became incorporated into much more wide-ranging and systematic systems for clinical accountability and standard setting. More comparative information was made available to managers and purchasers about the outcomes of clinical audit so that they could be better assured of the quality of the services that were being offered and purchased. From the mid-1990s, the Department of Health began a big educational and publicity drive around the concept of 'evidence-based medicine', publishing systematic meta-reviews of evaluative research literature on treatments and procedures, sponsoring special training courses and encouraging doctors to adopt current best practice.

Since 1999, NSFs (National Service Frameworks), NICE (National Institute for Clinical Excellence), which you read about in Chapter 2, and other central guidance, threaten to limit medical autonomy with national recommendations as to how services are to be configured, which treatments are approved as clinically efficacious and cost-effective and what standards of performance are expected. The clinical audit processes now have an expanded set of nationally defined requirements and standards to attain. From 2000, the **Commission for Health Improvement** (CHI) has acted like a national inspectorate to follow up compliance with these standards, making regular visits and immediate investigations if concerns have been raised about a Trust's performance and standardising key areas of medical practice.

Meanwhile, the professional status of medicine at a national level has been somewhat challenged by several well-publicised cases of professional negligence. In response, the General Medical Council (GMC) has tightened up on procedures whereby doctors can be investigated for incompetence as well as misconduct. Furthermore, as with other health-care professions, new proposals for 'revalidation' are being introduced to ensure that doctors' knowledge and skills are kept up to date throughout their careers (although at the time of writing in 2001, the British Medical Association and the GMC had not agreed how revalidation would be carried out).

While there has been no simple takeover of clinical power by management, central control has increased through the gradual and incremental tightening of a variety of direct and indirect mechanisms, which have constrained individual medical freedom and brought budgets, workflow and treatment quality under a much higher degree of co-ordination and control. The 21st century NHS Trust Chief Executive has medical and clinical directors to call on to 'cajole and persuade' medical staff, s/he can influence appointments, work plans and merit payments as far more information becomes available from internal clinical audit and quality procedures and from external standards and inspection from NICE and CHI activity. This information can be used to exert pressure on individual clinicians or directorates to improve performance and meet certain agreed targets and criteria. In this way, knowledge is power.

However, maintaining the confidence of the majority of clinicians is still essential for Chief Executive survival. Furthermore, the critical role of medical and clinical directors continues to ensure that doctors and their concerns are still central to the Trust's activities and they retain their influence over other professions. Likewise GPs, in their role of local commissioners of health services, have potentially more power than hospital directors. Thus, GPs continue to balance the two high-status activities of management and clinical practice.

3.5.3 Nursing — managers and managed

The dilemmas for nurses in their involvement in management are somewhat different from those facing doctors. At ward or unit level, many nurses are involved in the first-line management of more junior nurses and other staff. However, at this level there is face-to-face contact with patients and colleagues and a shared ideology around the imperatives of caring, which include the need to act as **patient advocates** by speaking up for patients and representing their interests. At more senior levels, nurses are involved in management with specific area or task responsibilities and there is a key dilemma of identity and commitment. The dilemma is that when nurse managers begin to take on the language and concerns of finance, performance and the detached systematic control of subordinates' work, it threatens the distinctive nursing identity gained after years of socialisation and colleagueship.

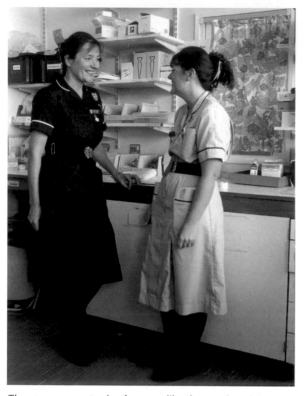

The management role of nurses, like the nursing sister featured here, places demands on their time and creates pressures that may be in conflict with their nursing role. (Photo: Mike Levers)

Nurse managers may continue to direct nursing standards and protocols, but continuing to perform nursing tasks on the ward would be to slot back into a subordinate and 'managed' role. It remains to be seen whether the return of the 'modern matron', a senior managerial figure with a strong, expanded professional responsibility at ward level, will help nurse managers to resolve this dilemma.

Part of the impact of the new approach to health management is the tendency to push responsibility down the line to professionals, so that they have to work within budgets and decide how to spend their time and how best to care for patients. The comments from nurses in a study by Michael Traynor (1999) into how nurse managers felt about their role emphasised a contrast between their competing concerns — practical patient care and the welfare of the staff — and the managerial responsibilities. One Staff Nurse reported:

> I feel that management are far too concerned with statistics and complicated paperwork, and as long as these are in order, they really aren't concerned about the patient's well-being. (Traynor, 1999, p. 143)

A Nurse Executive felt strongly that:

> (we) … actually have to be able to say very clearly to nurses what it is we expect of them within their current job, or within the resources that they have, so that they don't go around like headless chickens … and I suppose that is part of changing the culture of nursing slightly. (*ibid.*, p. 111)

The impact on front-line staff of managerial changes, coupled with growing consumer consciousness, are also brought out in a study carried out by Ellen Annandale (1996) on perceptions of risk held by nurses in an acute Hospital Trust. The threat of a patient complaint or even litigation was an ever-present worry, even for junior staff. It was felt that *The Patients' Charter* had encouraged a more critical attitude, and that 'covering your back' with extensive notes was a widespread defensive strategy.

> I am concerned because management won't back you up, and someone is always singled out to take the blame. (Staff Nurse) (Annandale, 1996, p. 428)

> It is very frustrating with poor staffing levels because you are responsible for the patient's care. You know it is dangerous potentially, but management refuses to accept this. When things go wrong you are left to pick up the pieces and take the blame and management wriggle out of responsibilities somehow. (Sister) (*ibid.*, p. 430)

● How does the management role affect the nursing profession in these accounts?

■ These nurses appear to be affected by an identity crisis that results from the conflicting relationships between being a nurse and being a manager. This impacts upon the unity of the profession as nurses on the front line feel more exposed and unsupported in their concern for direct patient care.

3.6 Dilemmas in managing primary care

Primary care has developed over the past 50 years, with GPs as independent contractors to the NHS initially becoming organised into group practices, then in the early 1990s taking on the role of fundholders. In 2000, they were grouped together into **Primary Care Groups** (PCGs), which will evolve into a smaller number of larger **Primary Care Trusts** (PCTs) by 2002, which will have more power and autonomy. PCG chairs were usually elected local GPs, but PCT chairs are appointed by the Secretary of State for Health. Chief Executive Officers (CEOs) of PCTs are selected through the same procedure as any hospital staff, using NHS personnel procedures. Other members of the PCT include at least one nurse representative, a lay member, a social services representative and a nominee from the district health authority.

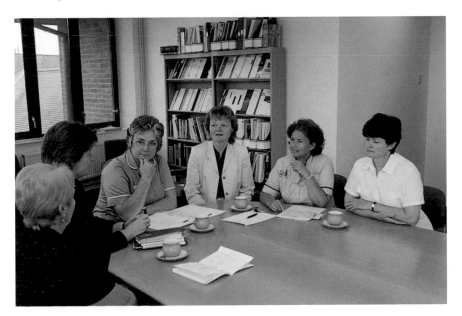

Primary Care Groups have evolved into increasingly autonomous and powerful gatekeepers of health-care provision. This is a weekly staff meeting of a PCG in Buckinghamshire. (Photo: Mike Levers)

Distinctive dilemmas continue to face professionals and managers within the new primary care framework. These new collective organisations of PCGs and PCTs offer attractions to managers and professionals in terms of extra resources and influence over health care, but there are considerable managerial and collaborative challenges to overcome before these benefits can be realised. The very process of setting up these groups, reorganising boundaries and applying for Trust status etc., is time-consuming and a distraction from on-going health issues. Managing a group of 'independent practitioners' and maintaining partnership arrangements with other local agencies, such as Social Services Departments, is full of complexities, and acting as both the providers and purchasers of health care has the potential to compromise managers in either of these roles and to threaten their relationship of trust with their patients. Consequently, the commissioning role which has been given to PCGs and PCTs means taking difficult and potentially unpopular decisions.

The PCTs will be responsible for both commissioning secondary care and providing a full range of primary care services. There will be only 50 PCTs for the whole of England, so they will cover large populations and have substantial budgets and responsibilities. Although GPs will continue to be important members of the Trust Board, they will have lost their position of being the controlling group. For busy GPs there must be a dilemma about whether to get drawn into these complex and time-consuming organisational activities at the price of neglecting their own practices.

Open University students should now read the article 'Improving NHS performance: human behaviour and health policy', originally published in 1999, by the health policy analyst Chris Ham. An extract appears in Davey, B., Gray, A. and Seale, C. (eds) *Health and Disease: A Reader* (Open University Press, 3rd edn 2001). As you read this, answer the following questions:

● (a) What are the key changes in management since the 1990s in the NHS, according to Chris Ham?

  (b) What does he consider to be the current 'preferred' model of management?

■ (a) Chris Ham suggests that there have been two key changes: the second way and the rise of third way. The second way was based on competition and empowerment, whereas the third way combined these aspects with central control, from which Ham lists such mechanisms as inspection, regulation and the publication of performance indicators.

  (b) Chris Ham suggests that there is still the potential for a 'third way' between bureaucratic and market-led styles, and one that allows for 'entrepreneurial managers and clinicians'.

The extension of the Trust concept to primary care has been crucial because it creates within primary care the key infrastructure of an 'enterprise'. The PCT is, first, a structure within which internal management can be exercised with objectives, controls, procedures, budgets and information flows. Secondly, the PCT can be subject to external control, evaluation, assessment and monitoring by NHS performance managers to ensure compliance with standards and policies. Ultimately, PCTs judged to be successful may be rewarded with extra resources and allowed to expand their scope and territory. Less successful PCTs can potentially be helped to improve, named and shamed, have their resources curtailed or even be taken over.

However, some commentators suggest that the workload and pressure of setting up the new organisations and carrying out the required tasks inevitably inflate the power, influence and responsibility of the full-time Chief Executives of PCTs and their staff. This strategy of creating groups of GPs has drawn them into a bigger management structure with greater budgetary and service responsibilities. PCTs in their turn will become substantial organisations with the capacity to take over, directly or through contracting, much of the work of community care Trusts and especially community nursing. The question remains of how the dilemma in managing primary care can be resolved by placing providers and purchasers into Trusts.

3.7 Conclusions — the inevitability of management?

Some commentators have suggested that it is impossible to manage a comprehensive, publicly funded, national health service and balance the increasing demands from new technological possibilities and rising consumer expectations. This tension may well lead to major policy changes which move towards the mixed-funding models of other Western societies.[6] But, in 2000 *The NHS Plan* explicitly rejected alternative funding methods as being more expensive, and celebrated a determination to make a 'modernised' NHS work. However, since the NHS is such a political concern to voters and politicians (as discussed in Chapter 1), it is likely that new management techniques will continue to be introduced, changed and modified. In this context, managers will continue to be subject to changing demands and to be faced with the need to resolve dilemmas by making difficult choices.

OBJECTIVES FOR CHAPTER 3

When you have studied this chapter, you should be able to:

3.1 Define and use, or recognise definitions and applications of, each of the terms printed in **bold** in the text.

3.2 Describe the tensions between local and central responsibility for managing the NHS.

3.3 Discuss the dilemmas that doctors and nurses face in their role as managers, and comment on differences between their spheres of influence.

3.4 Discuss the key dilemma that arises in the delivery of primary health care, from the tension between the commissioning of health services and the provision of primary and secondary health care.

[6] The unique funding of the NHS and the contrast with insurance-based health services in other Western countries is discussed in *Caring for Health: History and Diversity* (Open University Press, 3rd edn 2001), Chapter 9.

QUESTIONS FOR CHAPTER 3

1   (*Objective 3.2*)

Suggest some of the difficulties that arise in managing the relationship between the central and local levels of the NHS.

2   (*Objective 3.3*)

Pauline Miles is a ward sister on an acute surgical ward. The ward is short of staff and her annual budget for additional cover from staff brought in from a nursing agency is almost spent after only six months. Pauline wants to close beds on the ward because of the staff shortage, but has met with resistance from the surgical consultant who has a target set by hospital managers to reduce the elective surgery waiting list.

(a) What dilemmas does this raise for Pauline?

(b) Why might it prove more costly to keep beds open under these conditions?

(c) In the situation described, explain why nurses such as Pauline are likely to wield less influence than doctors such as the surgical consultant.

3   (*Objective 3.4*)

Primary Care Trusts acting as both the providers and commissioners of health care face a conflict of interest that is difficult to resolve. What are some of the potential effects of this conflict of interest on GPs?

CHAPTER 4

Dilemmas in community care

Study note for OU students

In Chapters 6 and 7 of *Caring for Health: History and Diversity* (Open University Press, 3rd edn 2001), you considered an analysis of the development of the concept of community care and an overview of more recent developments in health and community care partnerships. Taken together, they form the basis of this chapter's more focused exploration of community-care policy and practice and the associated dilemmas. The examination of health-care expenditure in Chapter 9 of that book is also useful reading for this chapter. You will also be introduced to some of the issues that relate to the role of formal and informal carers. The audiotape 'Who cares?' presents the views of formal and informal carers in the community and provides examples of their personal dilemmas.

You could also usefully read the article in *Health and Disease: A Reader* (Open University Press, 3rd edn 2001) written by the Sainsbury Centre for Mental Health entitled 'Being there', which describes the experience of being on an acute psychiatric ward.

This chapter was written by Bob Hudson, who is a principal research fellow at Nuffield Institute of Health in Leeds.

4.1 Introduction: defining terms

> To the politician it is a useful piece of rhetoric; to the sociologist it is a stick to beat institutional care with; to the civil servant it is a cheap alternative to institutional care which can be passed to the local authorities for action or inaction; to the visionary it is a dream of the new society in which people really do care; to social services departments it is nightmare of heightened expectations and inadequate resources to meet them. We are only just beginning to find out what it means to the old, the chronic sick and the handicapped. (Jones *et al.*, 1978, p. 114)

This quote from Kathleen Jones and colleagues about social care remains relevant, even though it was written in the late 1970s. Indeed, community care has remained ostensibly high on the social policy agenda of all governments since the mid-1950s, although much of the debate has centred upon issues of public policy such as finance, management and organisational structure. Despite this focus, the concept of **community care** continues to be poorly defined, and many of the tensions produced by such different understandings of what community means lead to dilemmas in the practice of community care.

The social relations of communities, and the ways in which these are bounded by such things as geographical location or membership, are subject to both prescriptive and descriptive interpretations. In terms of popular imagery, the notion of **community** represents warmth, intimacy and a settled group of people sharing both a set of values and a way of life that is often considered to be lacking today. But while it is recognised that there are some tightly knit communities in Britain, Meg Stacey, a leading sociologist, has advocated abandoning the term because it places expectations of support on family members, in particular women (Stacey, 1969). Although community support through social networks, sometimes called 'social capital',[1] is considered to be a key resource in protecting people's health, the role of care within the community often falls to the immediate family members.

Not only is the term *community* difficult to define but the term **care** also conveys different meanings. *Care* implies two things: a set of tasks and a relationship. For example it is possible to *care* about people who live at a great distance from us and also to provide *care* for someone through physical and emotional help and support. There is a social expectation in that it is thought to be 'good' to care for someone and, furthermore, detrimental to be uncaring. The role of caring is therefore underpinned by assumptions that produce expectations of care provision. The provision of community care is dependent upon an understanding of what it means in practical terms.

Despite the recognition that the term is unhelpful, the idea that there was some 'golden age' in which neighbours were bound together in small communities continues to dominate the thinking about what communities *ought* to be like and how they ought to function. Community is not just an idea, but also a place. The community, as a place where formal nursing and social care is given, has complex meanings attached to it. For example, there are different types of home for older people. These are registered according to who owns them and are either 'local

---

[1] A discussion of 'social capital' occurs in *World Health and Disease* (Open University Press, 3rd edn, 2001), Chapter 10, and in an article by its principal advocate, Richard Wilkinson, entitled 'The psychosocial causes of illness', in *Health and Disease: A Reader* (Open University Press, 3rd edn, 2001), which is optional reading for Chapter 9 of the current book.

authority', 'voluntary' (non-profitmaking) or 'private'. Residents are expected to contribute to the payment for their care according to their means. The size of these homes ranges from one to 500 residents, although the average-sized home houses about 30–40 residents, which means they often resemble institutions more than homes. They are also classified by their purpose and can be residential, nursing and dual-registered. This involves classifying the residents according to their social or nursing needs.

For example, the residents of all types of home can receive both care from a GP and hospital care. Only residents of residential homes are entitled to the routine provision of nursing care from community nurses in the community-home setting, although nursing-home staff can and do call upon specialist nurses for help and advice, even though they have qualified nurses on duty. In Scotland, nursing-home care is paid for by the health authority as a recognised part of NHS care and as an entitlement. This has raised the issue of who should pay for 'health' care.

The example of residential and nursing homes illustrates the complexity of community as a setting. It also suggests a lack of equity in the provision of health and social care. In particular, the reality of what actually constitutes a community impacts upon the quality and context of the care that is given to its often vulnerable members.

The reality of life in the community is that it includes both domestic and communal settings. Institutions that are considered to be part of the community are called 'homes', but often remain separate from the social relations of the community, sharing only the same geographic boundary. The residents of some homes, most commonly people with mental health problems, may not be accepted by the local community because of the stigma that is attached to their condition.

The formal provision of community care by local and health authorities, and the policy requirement that these authorities work together across health-care and social-care boundaries, has become the focus of many tensions. In attempting to solve the problem of separating health and social care, the expectation that people could work in partnership has created further dilemmas, which are the subject of the next section.

4.2 Dilemmas in community care

The notion of a golden age of the community creates an expectation of something that is difficult to translate into practice. How can society meet the public expectation of what care should be like when its definition is subject to political rhetoric and its practice is dynamic and changing?

The experience of care in the community is that it is often care *by* the community, usually the family, mostly by women. The increasing number of older people with care needs and the decreasing number of younger people available to satisfy them, and changes in family structures and work patterns, mean that there are fewer potential informal carers available. Clearly, without the necessary support, formal or otherwise, this will lead to increasing difficulty in providing care in the community. The dilemma here is how can care be provided in a way that is affordable yet non-exploitative, and acceptable to both the carers and those in need of care?

Even if there were enough informal carers able to provide care, would it be ethically justifiable to expect them to care, and do people want to be cared for by family members?

Should we expect the state and local government to provide full care to older people, people with learning disabilities, chronically ill and frail citizens in their own domestic homes, or should we continue to depend upon residential- and nursing-home care? In stark terms, the choice is between the exploitation of informal carers, who are mostly women, and an increasing amount of state funding for formal community care or for care provision by residential and nursing homes, which are seen by some as profiteering and institutions in disguise. Further, how are the boundary disputes between the health service and social services over 'who cares?' and 'who pays for it?' to be resolved? Who controls costs and sets standards for quality?

Finally, even if it can be argued that people who have difficulties that are socially unacceptable should live in the community, how are the views of the people in the vicinity to be valued? How are those individual rights and freedoms to be given priority when they are in conflict and one person's freedom erodes someone else's rights?

The tensions around these dilemmas have been reflected in the development of community-care policy, as you will see in the next section.

4.3   The development of community-care policy

Since the 1980s, three dimensions have structured the debate about the development of community-care policy, which has changed over time. These have been:

*   a shift in *location*: from institution to community;

*   a shift in *perspective*: of the value of community care;

*   a shift in *power*: from agencies and professions to users and carers.

4.3.1 A shift in location: from institution to community

Institutional care of chronically sick, disabled or frail older people only began in the middle of the nineteenth century. Before that time, parishes made provision for care of the 'sick poor' in their own homes, often by paying poor people locally to do the caring.

Since the 1980s many large hospitals that looked after mental health patients have closed, and the land has been sold for private development. Severals Hospital in Colchester, which housed 212 patients, was closed on 31 March 1999. (Photo: John Callan, Shout)

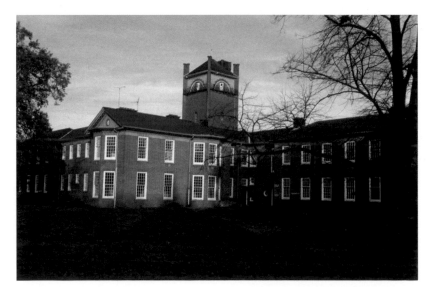

However, during the Victorian period there was an inexorable growth of institutions – in particular the 'poor law' workhouses, asylums for people deemed to be insane, and long-stay hospitals.[2] It was not until the early part of the twentieth century that the tide began to turn back towards some forms of community care, albeit on a modest scale. The Mental Deficiency Act of 1913, for example, contained provisions for the voluntary and statutory supervision of 'the mentally deficient' in the community, and the 1930 Mental Treatment Act recognised a growing movement for outpatient clinics. In the field of childcare, the Curtis Report (1946) recommended that preference be given to the care of children taken into care in ordinary families or small group homes, rather than large establishments. These developments were usually referred to as 'after care', with an assumption that hospitalisation was the central part of the intervention even if it was no longer the entirety. Questions about the need for the admission of adults to an institution were raised very slowly as the trend toward care in the community gained greater acceptance.

The real shift of emphasis in mental health-care provision came in 1961 when the Minister of Health, Enoch Powell, announced 'the run-down of the mental hospital'. With references to 'the defences we have to storm' and 'setting the torch to the funeral pyre', he announced that the country's 150 000 mental-hospital beds would be reduced to half that number by 1975.

In the 20 years or so following Enoch Powell's speech, much of the controversy over community care concerned the extent to which long-stay institutions were decreasing, the desirability of such a shift and the consequences of doing it. Although initially closures were limited, throughout the second half of the 1980s and through the 1990s, the old long-stay hospitals began to disappear. The process gathered momentum and 'deinstitutionalisation' was tacitly accepted as a general policy. Between 1980 and 1991, for example, the number of people with a learning disability living in long-stay NHS institutions in Britain fell from 56 000 to 30 000, and by 1997–98 this had been further reduced to around 12 000. In the case of mental illness, the number of in-patients fell from 150 000 in the 1950s, to 50 000 at the end of the 1980s and just under 38 000 by the end of 1997–98 (Department of Health, 1999a).

The concern about the effects of **institutionalisation** was part of the drive towards community care. People in institutions who have all their decisions made for them quickly lose control over most aspects of their life and often with this their self-confidence and ability to make decisions. However, while one problem might have been solved by changing location, these changes seemed to raise different concerns about the quality of life in the community, both for service users themselves and their informal carers.

4.3.2 A shift in perspective: the value of community care

In the 1970s, in the field of learning disability, a lobby formed from which a new philosophy of **normalisation** was born, which was based on the right to an 'ordinary life' and which included the right to live in the community and participate in community life (**social model of disability**).

---

[2] The history of workhouses and asylums is discussed in *Caring for Health: History and Diversity* (Open University Press, 3rd edn 2001), Chapters 1–4.

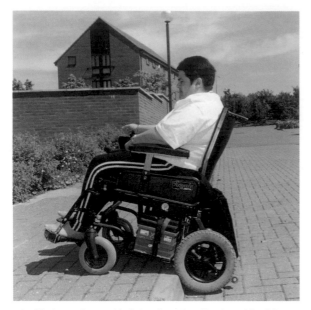

Disabled people would claim that they live in a 'disabling society'. (Photo: Mike Levers)

The practical implications of normalisation for community care are how services can be provided in a way that empowers individuals to attain these rights. The right balance between autonomy and paternalism is difficult to achieve in any context, particularly so with people who have been subjected to continuous professional power and control mostly in institutions, often by virtue of being labelled as 'disabled'.

Normalisation as a strategy is sufficiently general to apply to other groups covered by the policy of community care, notably older people, people with mental health problems and people with a physical disability, but in general these groups have been less powerful than the learning disability lobby. Moreover, as will be seen later, many current forms of support do not always measure up to the imperatives of normalisation.

Much of the debate over care in the community focuses on whether or not people with severe mental health problems are able to be treated in the community at all. Claims that institutional psychiatry has failed are in conflict with the continued need to provide in-patient services for people who are 'in crisis'. The best site for the treatment of people with these acute needs is likewise contested.

● Suggest what dilemma results from the public and media focus of community care on people with mental health problems who are considered to be a risk to others.

■ What is normalisation for one group is a lack of security for wider society. The rights of mental health-service users and the right of citizens to be safe are in direct conflict.

High-profile cases such as Dunblane, in which a man with a mental illness shot 16 pupils and their teacher in a school, and wounded 10 pupils and three staff members, attract a lot of media attention. It could be argued that such tragedies have fuelled a moral panic, which is a reaction against 'madness' in the community. It contributes to the need for society to keep itself safe from mental illness and therefore to keep unsafe people segregated from society and in institutions.[3]

These problems raise the concern of how control can be transferred from institutions to the community.

4.3.3 A shift in power: from agencies and professionals to users and carers

The transfer in power from organisations and professions towards services users is starker in the field of physical disability. This is because there has been a long-running difference of opinion about the nature of physical disability and its relationship to service provision.

[3] Evidence for this claim can be found in the case study on schizophrenia in *Experiencing and Explaining Disease* (Open University Press, 2nd edn 1996; colour-enhanced 2nd edn 2001), Chapter 6.

Normalisation has been criticised for its tendency to make the experiences of people with disabilities invisible. The argument is that, by moving the focus away from disabilities, people's needs are not met because they are not formally acknowledged. Furthermore, people accordingly become objects to be treated, changed, improved and made 'normal', while the physical and social environment is taken to be inflexible and unadaptable.

The way in which disability is defined impacts upon the care that is available in the community.

● Suggest why people with physical disability might have particular practical problems with normalisation.

■ People with physical disability are more likely to need equipment and physical adjustments to their homes to facilitate their independence. If their needs are not recognised, very basic amenities will not be made available.

From agencies to carers

The last two decades have witnessed a remarkable rise in recognition of the importance of informal care within the policy agenda, exemplified in the popularisation of the term **carer**.

At the turn of the twenty-first century, there were 5.7 million carers in Britain providing unpaid support to family members, partners or friends in need of care. Of these carers, 3.3 million (about 60 per cent) were women and 2.4 million (about 40 per cent) were men, of mostly middle age, from 45 to 64, although a notable number were children (between 20 000 and 50 000). The people they cared for also belonged to all age groups, with half of all carers caring for someone over 75 years old. Nearly half of all carers (49 per cent) were in full- or part-time paid employment, with 26 per cent retired and 25 per cent unemployed. Married older people in need of care were more likely to receive this care from their spouse (Department of Health, 2000b).

Figure 4.1 maps the detailed breakdown of the percentages of carers in the regions of the UK. The range of 11–17 per cent of the population who are carers is a graphic illustration of the high level of caring that takes place in the community by informal carers.

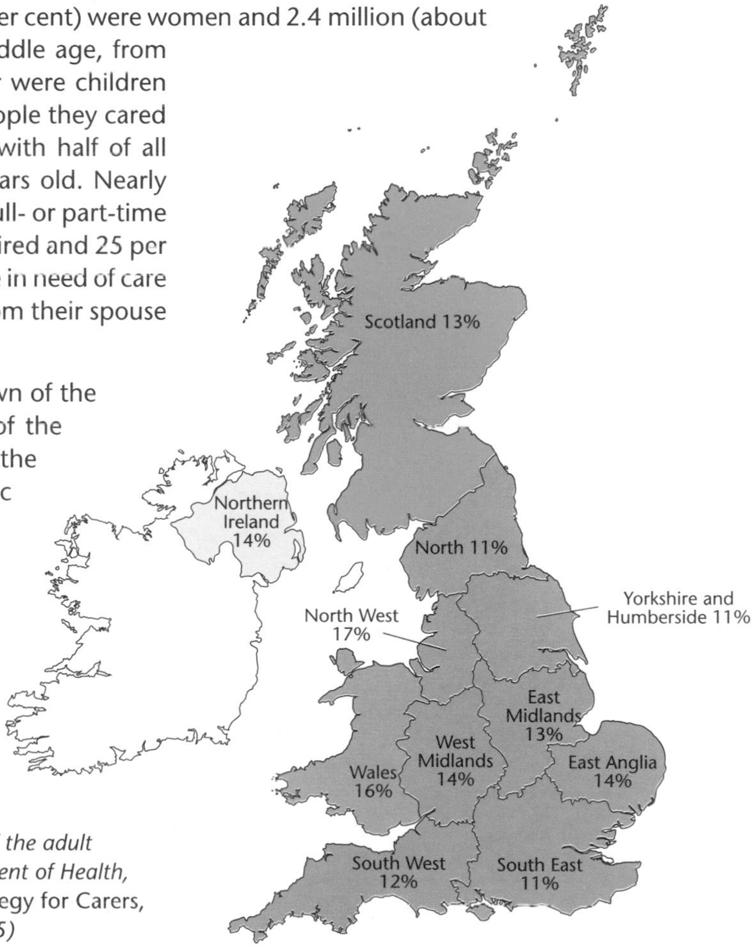

Scotland 13%

Northern Ireland 14%

North 11%

North West 17%

Yorkshire and Humberside 11%

East Midlands 13%

West Midlands 14%

East Anglia 14%

Wales 16%

South West 12%

South East 11%

Figure 4.1 *Map showing the percentage of the adult population who are carers. (Source: Department of Health, 2000b,* Caring about Carers: National Strategy for Carers, *2nd edn, The Stationery Office, London, p. 15)*

Figure 4.2 illustrates details of carers and cared-for in households in which caring involved more than eight hours per day.

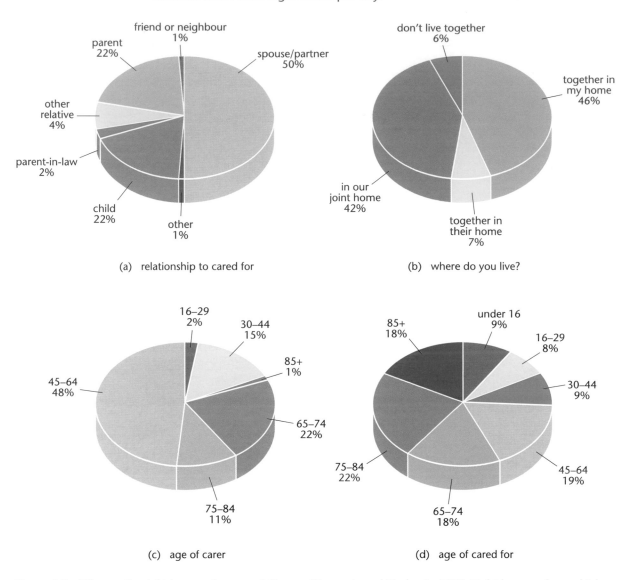

(a) relationship to cared for

(b) where do you live?

(c) age of carer

(d) age of cared for

Figure 4.2   *Who are the eight hours a day carers? (Source: Warner, L. and Wexler, S., 1998,* Eight hours a day and taken for granted, *The Princess Royal Trust for Carers, London, Figures 4, 5, 6 and 7, p. 9)*

- What does Figure 4.2 tell you about 'who cares?', where the cared-for person needs eight hours or more support per day?

- Almost all carers (98 per cent) were related to the cared-for person (50 per cent were partners or spouses), and lived with the person they looked after (94 per cent). Thus, caring is a 'round the clock' responsibility, usually within one's own household.

- What do the ages of the carers tell you about the carers?

- Many of the carers are older people, who may benefit from being cared for themselves.

(Open University students should now listen to Side 1 of the audiotape 'Who cares?', in which a small group of informal carers discuss their experience of caring.)[4]

● What is the main frustration expressed by the carers in the group?

■ They all wanted to care for their family member but did not feel that they had enough support to enable them to do so in the way that they wished.

What is clear from the audiotape is that community care places a burden of care on close family. Care in the community can isolate those in receipt of care and also their carers and limit their choices and control. Furthermore, the burden placed upon families in providing informal care can be heavy and may subsequently reduce their ability to make use of social networks and support systems, because so much of their time and energy is taken up with caring.

The increasing acknowledgement by policy-makers that most care for older and disabled people is provided by their families has been seen as a highly cost-effective strategy. It is a way of maximising the input of carers through the judicious use of formal support, which has been seen as a highly cost-effective strategy, although there has also been increased recognition of the needs and interests of carers *per se*. Carers accordingly featured in several policy initiatives of the 1990s, such as the Carers (Recognition and Services) Act 1996 which entitled carers to receive a separate assessment of their needs, though crucially it did not entitle them to resources. In 1999, the government published further proposals on a National Carers Strategy (Department of Health, 2000b), covering the setting of new standards, additional money to fund respite care and a second pension for carers.

4.4 The changing policy context of community care: public funding

In Chapters 2 and 3 of this book, you read about the separation of purchasing and provision of health care. Social care was also affected, and in 1990 the NHS and Community Care Act (Department of Health, 1990) made local authority social services responsible for the organisation and funding of community care, but it replaced traditional public sector bureaucracies by what has been termed **government by the market**. The intentions were that provider competition would supply incentives for greater responsiveness to the needs of consumers, while being attentive to cost and quality. At the same time, health-care and social-care boundaries were being blurred.

The 1990 Community Care Act was implemented in 1993 and local authorities were given the freedom to spend money on either institutional or non-institutional care. But the '85 per cent rule' required them to spend 85 per cent of this money on providers in the independent sector. The shift in location from institutions to communities was a direct result of this change in social security payments.

---

[4] This audiotape has been recorded for undergraduates studying this book as part of an Open University course. An article by Michael Young and Lesley Cullen, 'The carer at home', further illustrates this theme; it appears in *Health and Disease: A Reader* (Open University Press, 3rd edn, 2001).

Costs of support from the Department of Social Services to residents in all types of residential and non-residential home grew from £39 million to £2.57 billion between 1982 and 1993. As mentioned earlier, it is in the provision of nursing and residential care where the distinction between health care and social care is extremely difficult to make. Until 1980, private provision in residential and nursing homes remained small. Social services departments came into existence in 1971 based upon an implicit understanding that the **personal social services**, defined as services that enable people to function as independently as possible in their own home and include household tasks, personal care and support to informal carers, would be both state funded and state provided; the profit motive was felt to be incompatible with the provision of care for vulnerable people.

Between 1970 and 1998, local authority and voluntary residential-care provision had fallen by two-thirds and the private sector places by more than four-fold (Hardy and Wistow, 1999). Table 4.1 shows the proportions spent on different client groups by local authorities in England on personal social services in 1998–99.

Table 4.1 Gross expenditure by local authorities in England on personal social services by client group, 1998–99, in millions of pounds.

	Elderly	Children	Learning disability	Physical disability	Mental health	Other	Total
HQ costs	–	–	–	–	–	149	149
area officers/senior managers	103	161	26	29	28	–	348
care management/ care assessment	329	505	76	101	126	–	1 136
residential care	3 180	724	838	218	224	–	5 184
non-residential care	1 605	1 074	555	402	186	–	3 822
other	–	–	–	–	–	208	208
Total	5 216	2 465	1 495	750	564	357	10 847

Source: Department of Health (2000) *Health and Personal Social Services Statistics,* Section E: Expenditure, Table E5, accessed on 26 July 2001 from: www.doh.gov.uk/HPSSS/INDEX/HTM.

Over a ten-year period, the increase in the private sector homes reflected the decrease in NHS long-stay care. The number of long-stay NHS beds fell by 54 per cent between 1970 and 1998. This was a dramatic shift from publicly funded care free at the point of delivery, to private sector care funded by residents or from means-tested local authority support.

● From Table 4.1, what proportion of the personal social-services budget was spent on older people? Of the money spent on older people, what proportion was spent on residential as opposed to non-residential care?

■ Almost half of the total budget was spent on older people, and of that twice as much was spent on residential as on non-residential care.

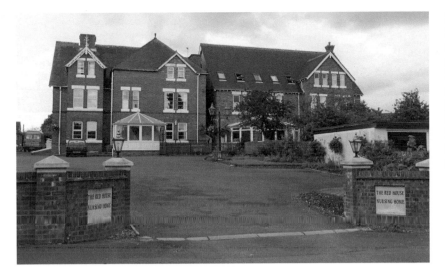

From the 1980s, the increased demand for private residential and nursing homes meant that many domestic houses were converted. They were not purpose-built and were often poorly designed for the provision of care to older people. Disabled access to and within homes such as the one featured here is a particular problem. (Photo: Mike Levers)

4.5 Partnerships in community care

The shift to partnerships and joint working between the health service and local authority social services departments has meant a shift of focus to the boundary between health care and social care. Legislation of the late 1990s provided new structures with which the rhetoric and the reality could be matched. There was a very close relationship between the proposed changes to the NHS and the organisation of social care, respectively. The Government announced its proposals in the White Paper called *Modernising Social Services* (Department of Health, 1998a), parts of which carried important implications for health care and social care relationships. **Continuing care** services are health services provided outside hospital settings by the NHS, usually for people with chronic, degenerative and age-related diseases. The aim is to do this by collaborating with local authorities and other organisations inside and outside the NHS. The distinction from community care is in terms of who is the lead provider and depends upon how care needs are classified as being either health or social ones. Demands for health and social-care agencies to work in an integrated way do not take account of the reality that they are distinctly different organisations. In many ways, different organisational activities are more difficult obstacles that have to be overcome. Furthermore, joint commissioning is a new way of addressing the old problems of the fragmentation and inflexibility of community care.

4.5.1 Seamless services?

Primary Care Groups (PCGs) were included in the management of care across boundaries between health care and social care, further emphasising the goal of meeting health and social-care needs through **joined-up working**. Although Section 10 of the 1973 NHS Act had placed health and local authorities under a statutory duty to cooperate, this duty was general rather than specific, and was not supported by formal accountability arrangements. The joint commissioning by PCGs was part of the new formal arrangement after 1997 (see Section 4.5.2). Conversely, the White Paper *Modernising Social Services* revisited this type of legislative partnership and proposed a new statutory 'duty of partnership' to require NHS bodies and local authorities to 'work together for the common good'.

4.5.2 Partnerships in action

Many of the proposals in *Modernising Social Services* stem from the discussion document, *Partnership in Action* (Department of Health, 1998b), which was published slightly earlier and which specifically addressed the interface between the NHS and social services. The paper identified the need for joint working at the following levels.

Strategic planning between health-care and social-care agencies, which requires them to plan jointly for the medium term, and share information about how they intend to use their resources towards the achievement of common goals.

In lead commissioning, the sharing of health authority and local authority boundaries is far from straightforward and is the arena of many disputes. One simple dispute involves the reality that local authorities, health authorities and PCGs all serve different populations. The suggestion that PCGs will typically serve populations of around 100 000 means that for smaller local authorities they will share the same geographical area as the PCG, whereas larger local authorities may have up to ten PCGs in or on the borders of their area. Primary Care Trusts (PCTs), which will evolve from PCGs by 2004, combine several population groups but again the boundaries with social service areas are not necessarily shared.

The question of whether it is possible to commission services more effectively and efficiently against the background of demographic changes and increasing demands for complex care will be difficult if not impossible to evaluate.

Regardless of how services are purchased or funded, the key objective of 'partnership in action' is that the user receives a coherent integrated package of care. The document *Partnership in Action* saw several fresh opportunities at the service provision level: the emerging PCTs, and the experiences gained from special initiatives, such as the 'winter pressures' money, which is extra funding to be used in community care to avoid hospital admissions if possible. In the particular case of older people, the government required that a framework was in place for multidisciplinary assessment of community health and acute-care settings, where local authorities would be required to spend part of their funding in support of rehabilitation and recuperation facilities.

However, there is more to partnerships than those between professional bodies. Some attempts have been made to include local citizens in local policy decisions on community care, but carers often feel excluded.

● In Side 1 of the audiotape 'Who cares?', Open University students heard informal carers talk about their experience of 'care in the community'. What was the carers' experience of joined-up working?

■ The informal carers expressed many concerns, which included being expected to provide most of the care for their relative, without adequate payment for doing so and not being able to access health-care and social-care resources effectively for their relative and themselves. They also claimed that professional carers failed to recognise them as part of the care team and dismissed both their contribution and their personal needs.

The main barriers to working across boundaries are the potential difficulties in how the relationship of power is shared between health and social services. The problem of who does what and who pays the cost, and establishing systems of effective communication, act as further barriers to effective joined-up working.

● Open University students should now listen to Side 2 of the audiotape 'Who cares?', which provides accounts by two teams of health professionals in the community. As you do so, answer the following questions: (a) What are the communication problems of both teams? (b) What level of support does the paediatric home-care team provide? (c) What concerns about resources does each team express?

■ (a) Paul, from the paediatric home-care team, expressed concerns about the poor level of understanding by GP surgeries of the role of the team. Marianne, from the same team, also described the difficulty of managing effective communication with many different hospitals. Members of the primary-care team complained about poor levels of written and verbal communication at the time of hospital discharge, although Fatimah (the midwife) found that this was resolved by the use of patient-held records in maternity care. Finally, Julian (the GP) contrasted this with the potential for new systems of electronic communication to increase the speed and amount of information available.

(b) The paediatric home-care team provide both practical and emotional support to families. Marianne described their liaison role, while Alison and Sian described the need of families for emotional support.

(c) Julian in the primary-care team discussed the problems of not being able to get people admitted to hospital because of 'blocked beds'. Both Julian and David (the community nurse) agreed that informal carers are vital to providing adequate care in the community, implying that resources would not be adequate without these 'free inputs'. Marianne and Alison of the paediatric home-care team expressed the need for respite care for the families they looked after, but did not have the resources to provide it.

The terms of involvement in consultation can reflect historical relationships of power and expertise so that not all parties are considered to be equal. Likewise, developing a relationship of trust requires people to transcend old barriers to working together and that takes time. The problems of measuring outcomes and agreeing what is most desirable can be a source of conflict between those involved and can also result in disputes about who is responsible for what care, who funds what and what are the care priorities.

The dilemma of how to involve people as equal partners across organisational boundaries makes power-sharing seem more of the rhetoric than the reality.

Increasing agency flexibility

A pilot study conducted to evaluate the purchasing of community care concluded the following:

> Strong policy guidance will be needed on the involvement of users, carers and voluntary agencies in the development of plans and on the importance of developing CCC (Community and Continuing Care) services (which may otherwise retreat down a long list of things to do by the newly formed groups). [...] The primary care organisations may need control over resources or other levers or incentives if they are to achieve true partnerships with social services and together achieve lasting change. (Wyke *et al.*, 1999, p. 406)

The Department of Health guidelines *Partnership in Action* highlight the need for further action and suggest three proposals for allowing more flexibility between agencies. The guidelines promote work between health and other agencies, such as housing, the probation service, the police and the voluntary sector.

- First, the legalisation of **pooled budgets** allows health and social services to pool their resources to commission and provide services in a way that would be accessible to both partners in the joint arrangements. Unlike the current position, the pooled resource would lose its health or social-services identity and be available for either type of support.

- Secondly, **lead commissioning**, in which one authority takes the lead in commissioning the range of services for a particular group on behalf of both agencies. Learning-disability and mental-health client groups are cited as areas of provision where this could be usefully applied. Such an arrangement could only flourish in a collaborative relationship that is characterised by a high degree of mutual respect and trust.

- And finally, the suggestion of more **integrated provision** and allowing health and social-services agencies to take on at least some of each other's functions.

4.5.3 Modernising social services

The White Paper *Modernising Social Services* (Department of Health, 1998a) adds to this agenda in a number of ways.

In arguing for a more accessible service, it espouses the 'one-stop-shop' model (perhaps better termed the 'first-stop-shop') to ensure that an approach to one agency will automatically trigger contributions from partner agencies as required.

A more significant measure, however, is the way that *Modernising Social Services* firmly grasps the importance of making partnership-working conditional upon access to resources. The main vehicle for this is through the pooled budgets of the £1.3 billion of new money contained in the Social Services Modernisation Fund, and in particular two 'Promoting Independence' grants — the Partnership Grant and the Prevention Grant — which between them total almost £750 million over a three-year period up to 2001–02. The larger of the two, the Partnership Grant, fosters partnership between health and social services. It promotes independence for service users as an objective of adult social services, with a particular emphasis upon improving rehabilitation services. The Prevention Grant focuses more upon developing preventive strategies to target people most at risk of losing their independence.

It seems that while the rhetoric of joint working and collaboration have been pushed forward by policy directives of central government, practice has shown that partnerships cannot be so easily imposed. The next section considers the outcomes of this for service users.

4.6   What has been achieved for users and carers?

So far in this chapter, we have indicated that a great deal has changed in the way services are organised and delivered in the community. Next, we give a very brief account of some of the current concerns relating to the four main client-service groupings: older people, people with learning difficulties or physical disabilities; and those with mental health problems.

4.6.1 Older people

The dilemma in providing community-care services to older people lies in the choice between targeting a smaller group who are most in need of care or providing diluted care to everyone with care needs.

In Figure 4.3, data collected by the Department of Health on the number of visits to households in England to provide personal social services show that, while costs for this provision have risen, the distribution of care has changed.

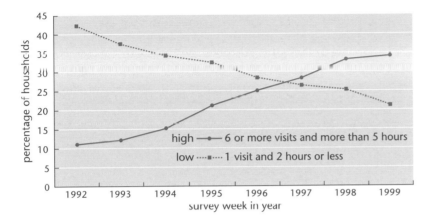

Figure 4.3 *Intensity of home help/home care, by percentage of households visited, in England in a survey week in each year between 1992 and 1999. (Source: Department of Health (1999)* Community Care Statistics 1999: Home Help/Home Care Services, England, *The Stationery Office, London, Figure 2, p. 5)*

● What is the most striking feature of Figure 4.3?

■ There is a steady trend from low- to high-intensity provision of home help and care between 1992 and 1999.

During the survey week in September 1999, an estimated 2.7 million contact hours were provided to around 424 000 households. Compared with 1998, this represents an increase in the number of contact hours of almost 3 per cent and a fall in the number of households receiving home help/home care of 5 per cent. This suggests that local authorities are providing more intensive services for a smaller number of service users.

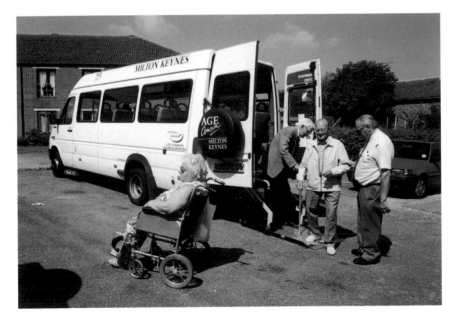

Older people arrive by transport at their local day centre. Day centres are one form of care provision that allows people to continue to live in their own homes. (Photo: Lionel Gretch)

The dilemma of providing more intensive services for fewer people or providing less intensive services for more is clearly demonstrated in Figure 4.3.

However, unlike earlier patterns of activity, this shift towards domiciliary and day care has been accompanied by what is being described as **higher service intensity** or targeting of those in the greatest need. Since 1993, this has generally meant an increase in the number of households provided with five hours or more of home-care services at the expense of those receiving what is termed 'low level care' of two hours or less per week. Since 1992, there has been a 9 per cent drop in the number of *households* receiving home-care services and a 56 per cent increase in the *contact hours* provided.

● What is the potential effect of concentrating services on people with greater care needs?

■ Ignoring people in lesser need of care can demote their independence, reduce their protection and lower standards, producing the opposite of the claimed objectives. A reduced level of support also puts pressure on informal carers to provide support to people or can produce the need for them to pay privately for these services in the short term. In the longer term it can mean that people decide to opt for residential care.

The following example from a study into the health needs of older people illustrates the limitations of the highest level of support that people can receive.

A study by Komaromy *et al.* (1999) revealed that even the most intensive care fell short of the high level of care and long hours that were needed. In 1994, in the North West of England, a community-based total-care team was set up to work closely with social-service care-managers, hospital and community staff to provide a precise assessment and ongoing review of the continuing care needs of older people, that is care that will be ongoing until the person dies, although the end of life might be unpredictable. A total-care team in this project provided care in domiciliary settings for people with high dependency needs that matched the criteria for nursing-home admission. Because the demand was so high, the team could cope with the care of only a small number of people. It was at first envisaged that the scheme would have an equal balance of input from social service and health support, but the main input of care was from the health authority. Care provision remained largely dependent upon the support of informal carers because the most intensive care that the team could provide was four visits per day and no cover at night. Even though the provision of continuing care in domestic settings was thought to be cheaper and more 'desirable' for patients, the health authority was constrained by resources.

4.6.2 People with learning disabilities, and issues of advocacy

The trends described earlier in this chapter have resulted in a significant improvement in service standards. For example, a recent investigation into services for adults by the Social Services Inspectorate (1998) praised the improvements that had taken place over the previous decade and noted that sound principles, along normalisation lines, had been developed, which emphasised independence, respect for users and community presence.

The following account is from Sheena Rolph, an educationalist who (at the time of writing in 2001) worked at the Open University as a research fellow. She carried out a study of the history of transition from institutional care to the community for people with learning disabilities; the following extract comes from her report.

People with learning disabilities are now beginning to talk and write about their lives, often challenging assumptions and stereotypes, as well as contributing rich new information about different experiences of community care.

For example, Jean's experience of what she regarded as community care in the 1960s was life in a NHS hostel after many years in an institution. In a conference presentation, Jean remembered her first few weeks in the hostel as, 'Heaven, absolute heaven ... I couldn't believe it. I was out. The doors were not locked'.

Eventually, in the mid-1970s with the national moves towards greater de-institutionalisation and normalisation, she moved to a small group home and then, in 1982, to a warden-run flat. She says about these transitions:

'The hostel was like your own home, but then I made another step forwards instead of backwards, I went to M. Road (the group home) and from there to B. Road with two wardens (the flat). We all (six friends) lived in flats in B. Road. R. was the warden there and she was very good because she got us all outings, we used to go to the pub, out in the minibus, have birthday parties. I made a lot of friends where I'm living now. It was easy, and I met a lot of people through my work'.

Contemporary rhetoric has tended to polarise institutional care and community care for people with learning difficulties at opposite ends of a scale, and has declared the latter to be superior to the former, despite evidence that it can be just as controlling and institutional. There are various degrees of community care, some still linked quite closely with institutional care, others enabling greater independence. Definitions of community care are therefore inevitably more complex and contradictory than is sometimes imagined. There are often many borders to cross, not one alone and several transitions to manage. (Rolph, 2000)

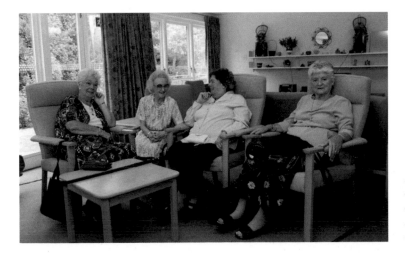

For many people who live in the community, the reality is living in a community home, which might carry many of the disadvantages of institutional care. (Photo: Lionel Grech)

Advocacy

As a social movement, advocacy started its history in the late 1960s with people with learning disabilities, and achieved full recognition in 1987 through the formation of the Advocacy Alliance. By this time, the advocacy movement included all groups such as older people, people with mental health problems, deaf and deaf/blind people. The requirement to involve users in the 1986 Disabled Persons' Act, the 1989 Children Act (Children Scotland Act) and the 1990 NHS and Community Care Act has resulted in a proliferation of advocacy projects.

Dorothy Atkinson, an Open University expert in this area, claims that **advocacy** for others can be distinguished into three main types (Atkinson, 1999):

- **Citizen advocacy**, a one-to-one relationship between client and a volunteer to provide support through friendship, spokepersonship and help in obtaining services.
- **Peer advocacy**, in which the advocate has some personal experience of the disability.
- **Children's advocates**, who are either volunteers as independent visitors or paid professional advocates.

She further highlights categories of people who do not have access to advocacy and includes people who are living in social isolation in the community, either in residential or non-residential care. Many professionals see themselves as advocates for their clients, but this raises a problem.

● What is a key disadvantage to using an advocate who is employed by the NHS or local authority?

■ Advocates might find that the interests of their client conflict with those of their employing authority.

But there is also a dilemma because professionals might be best placed to understand the client's needs and the details of their previous history and present circumstances. Independent advocates, however, might find it more difficult to influence the service providers and achieve outcomes for their clients.

It is clear that care in the community for people with learning and other disabilities has many problems. The slow speed of change and the transfer of institutional practices into community facilities have added to the problems that surround the lack of clear definitions of what community and care mean in reality.

4.6.3 People with a physical disability

In contrast to other service users, the area of physical disability has not been the subject of major policy changes such as the closure of long-stay institutions, and the majority of people with physical impairments are older people for whom disability is frequently seen as one aspect of ageing. Younger disabled people are not recognised as a separate group with specific needs and, in this sense, have been excluded from comparable policy imperatives.

Again, unlike services for older people and those with a learning disability, there has been a lesser degree of interagency conflict over responsibility for the support of and funding for physically disabled people. In part, this simply reflects the low level of long-stay provision within the NHS compared with that for other groups, but there are still areas of conflict over services. A particularly unhelpful distinction has been made between 'aids to daily living', such as wheelchairs and access ramps (a social-services responsibility) and 'nursing aids' such as incontinence pads and prostheses (an NHS one). This division of service is now often seen as one that can benefit from a joint-commissioning approach. As in the case of older people though, the tension between nursing and social care is increasing as the pressure to dismantle this artificial distinction increases.

In contrast to older people and people with a learning disability, expenditure on services for physically disabled people is weighted towards day care rather than residential care. This reflects attempts to maintain younger disabled people at home. The Royal Commission on Long-Term Care (1999), for example, notes that in England for each younger disabled person in a care home there are 14 households with a younger disabled person receiving home care. The comparable ratio for older people is nearer to two in a care home for every five households with home care, which reflects the strong emphasis on the community as the best place for younger people.

4.6.4 People with mental health problems

As in the case of people with learning difficulties, the mental health spotlight has turned away from institutions towards the effectiveness of community support. The release of large numbers of patients from mental hospitals from the 1960s onwards is felt to have caused significant problems both for former patients and for the communities that become their new homes. Manning and Shaw (1999) point out that adequate community services have often been unavailable to former patients, a large percentage of whom do not receive services or lose contact with services altogether. This occasionally culminates in highly publicised incidents, such as the cases in the 1990s of Ben Silcock, who climbed into the lions' den at London Zoo, and Graham Clunis, who stabbed Jonathan Zito to death in the London Underground. Such events put much pressure on governments to ensure that public safety is not compromised by community care programmes and has resulted in policy changes to assert greater control over people with severe mental illness.

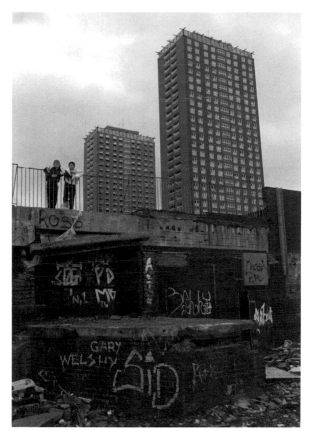

But people with mental health problems have always been subject to legislation which restricts their liberty. The Mental Health (Patients in the Community) Act 1996 requires patients subject to supervised discharge to abide by the terms of a care plan. This would mean that people who refused to take prescribed medication could be treated against their will, possibly in their homes. This proposal has united such diverse groups as Survivors Speak Out, Mind, and the Royal College of Psychiatrists in opposition to any move towards compulsory treatment outside of hospital.

People with mental health-care needs or with a history of mental illness often have difficulty gaining employment. Living on a reduced income for some people means living in areas that are deprived and this can lower their sense of self-esteem. (Photo: Jess Hurd/Report Digital)

The Minghella report, which evaluated the effectiveness of providing 24-hour psychiatric emergency care for people with mental health crises, answers the question of why people get referred to the psychiatric emergency team by claiming:

> The two largest categories were 'onset or relapse of psychotic symptoms' and 'risk of or actual harm to self or others'. This latter category included people displaying aggressive behaviours including setting light to furniture or threatening to harm themselves or others. Only one person in the sample actually harmed himself. This man had been accused of sexually abusing a young woman in his family; he took an overdose and attempted to throw himself in front of a car. It seems that the perceived threat or risk of harm to self or others was greater than actual harm. (Minghella *et al.*, 1999, p. 37)

● What key difficulty does this example highlight for the rights of mental health-service users?

■ As discussed in Section 4.3.2, one of the issues is the need to balance the rights of people with mental health problems against the need to protect the public from harm.

Care in the community for people with acute mental-health problems is rare, and most of the funds for acute care remain committed to acute psychiatric in-patient wards. Out-of-hours care, which offers a community alternative to in-patient admissions, is sadly lacking.

● What is the most likely consequence of the lack of appropriate care?

■ Many patients stay longer than necessary on acute wards through lack of alternatives.

Furthermore, the Sainsbury Centre for Mental Health, which provides research, training and service development for mental health-service users, claims that discharge from acute wards is often unplanned, with inadequate involvement of community staff, patients and carers. The threat of harm from people with mental health problems appears to outweigh the reality, and further highlights the complexity of managing care in the community when it is subject to so many tensions and dilemmas. Open University students might want to read the article 'Being there' in *Health and Disease: A Reader* (Open University Press, 3rd edn 2001), which describes the experience of being in hospital from the point of view of psychiatric in-patients.

4.7   Rhetoric and reality of community care

This section concludes the discussion of the dilemmas in community care. Two questions remain, which only time can answer:

- Is the gap between rhetoric and reality too wide to be bridged?
- Will the ideological divisions between interagency partnership and the market approaches to resource allocation continue to prevent the provision of any workable solutions?

The White Paper *Caring for People* (Department of Health, 1989) emphasised the importance of competition, privatisation and firmer monitoring, as well as better measurement of quality and some degree of partnership working – quite a tall order upon which to deliver. The Labour government elected in 1997 placed more emphasis upon partnership working, while, at the same time, retaining major elements of previous policy with little likelihood of the private sector losing its dominant provider role in institutional care.

Whatever the political persuasion determining policy decisions, the rhetoric of community care is based on an appeal to an imaginary supportive community and expectations of care from informal carers. Whether or not it is better for people to be cared for in the community varies between individuals and over time. The rhetoric is enshrined in economic and policy initiatives and is ideologically driven. For some people, the move to community care is a liberating experience, whereas for others it has hardly been distinguishable from the constraints of institutional life.

4.7.1 The future of community care

From the organisational point of view, there are changes in the way in which local government is being reformed. There are also possible changes arising from pressure upon community-care agencies to work together more closely. Primary Care Groups, and even more so, Primary Care Trusts, are likely to lead to a range of experiments with integrated structures combining social services, community health services and primary health care services. These changes, further encouraged by the new flexibilities, could encompass integrated working at strategic, commissioning and service delivery levels. Perhaps once such integrated arrangements begin to take hold, they could be based on what people need in the way of a better quality of life.

More pressing is the question of who will provide that care and at what cost. Dilemmas of community care have persisted over time despite attempts to address some of the key underlying difficulties. This chapter has considered some of the reasons for this continuation and has provided personal accounts of the experience of caring. As the debate continues, it will be helpful to ask what are the continuities and what are the changes? Are changes in community care merely rhetorical or have they addressed the real needs of a better quality of life for people and how community care can be constricted to effectively deliver this?

OBJECTIVES FOR CHAPTER 4

When you have studied this chapter, you should be able to:

4.1 Define and use, or recognise definitions and applications of, each of the terms printed in **bold** in the text.

4.2 Identify and describe the main dilemmas that arise from the delivery of community care.

4.3 Discuss the meaning of the term 'community care', and distinguish between the rhetoric and the reality of the experience of care in the community, including the point of view of informal carers.

4.4 Distinguish between the different issues of living in the community for the client groups of older people, people with physical disabilities, people with learning difficulties and mental health-service users.

QUESTIONS FOR CHAPTER 4

1   (*Objectives 4.2 and 4.3*)

Lucy is an 86-year-old woman who has been widowed for 12 months and has become increasingly depressed. She depends upon her neighbours for support with practical jobs like gardening and shopping, and her daughter at the weekends to help her with cooking meals and cleaning. She is considering going into a residential home, but is afraid of losing her own home, although she does not want to be a burden on her daughter. What aspects of the organisation of domiciliary support increase the likelihood that Lucy will enter residential care?

2   (*Objective 4.3*)

How might the meaning of the terms 'community' and 'care' impact on the reality of caring in the community?

3   (*Objectives 4.3 and 4.4*)

Sally lives in a community home for people with mental health problems. She has been trying to live independently for some months but her attempts have met with some resistance. Part of the concern about Sally living alone is the fact that she does not always take her medication and is prone to bouts of severe mood swings. What dilemmas does this raise for Sally and her formal carers?

C H A P T E R 5

Divisions in health-care labour

Study notes for OU students

This chapter builds on the discussion of health care in Chapters 5–7 of *Caring for Health: History and Diversity* (Open University Press, 3rd edn, 2001), which dealt with the historical context of the division of health work, the establishment of professional boundaries, the relative status of different professions and the impact of NHS changes upon the role of 'caring'. Based on these understandings, the chapter raises the dilemmas produced by the size, scope and divided nature of NHS employment.

During your study of this chapter you will be asked to read two articles — the first by Celia Davies is entitled 'Professionalism and the conundrum of care', and the second by Lesley Doyal and Ailsa Cameron, entitled 'Professions allied to medicine: continuity and change in a complex workforce', both of which can be found in *Health and Disease: A Reader* (Open University Press, 3rd edn 2001).

The audiotape 'Who cares?', which you listened to in the previous chapter, is also relevant and provides accounts of caring in the community by informal and professional carers.

This chapter was written by Carole Thornley who is a Senior Lecturer in Industrial Relations at Keele University.

5.1   Introduction: dilemmas in health work

The NHS employs around one million people in the UK and is one of the largest employers in Europe. The workforce includes highly trained and specialised medical staff, registered and non-registered nursing staff, technical, administrative, clerical and ancillary staff. These workers are employed in a wide variety of settings, from acute hospitals to learning disability and from community to family health services. 'Formal' health care in the UK is organised by the state and public sector, mainly through institutional arrangements, with other formal provision being made by the private and voluntary sectors. However, such formal arrangements are underpinned by an even larger 'informal' workforce of carers of at least 5.2 million people.

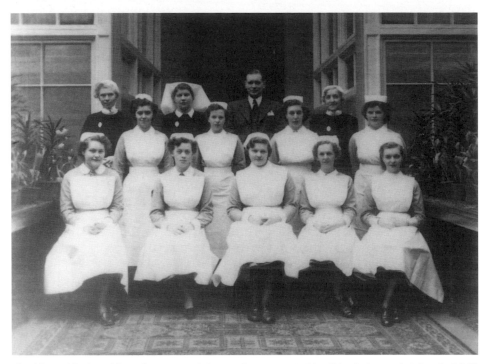

The hierarchical position of nurses and doctors is represented by this photograph taken in 1951 at Western Infirmary, Glasgow. The uniform serves as a powerful visual representation of the division of labour and demarcates status and position. (Photo: Royal College of Nursing Archives)

5.1.1   Labour specialism or labour division?

The sheer size and complexity of the NHS workforce can sometimes obscure the fact that there is still **division of labour** — a distinct hierarchy by class, gender and ethnicity (and associated pay rates), which closely resembles work organisation and wider inequalities in the private sector and reflects the historical roots of this division.

A key focus of this chapter is the way in which the modern NHS workforce, and the division of labour within it, have been shaped by conflicting forces: attempts by government and management to 'manage'; efforts by the (divided) representatives of health-care labour to obtain equitable reward and treatment and professional status; and public and electoral concerns and pressures. These forces have, of course, been both reflected in and influenced by wider changes in employment norms and trends in an advanced capitalist economy.

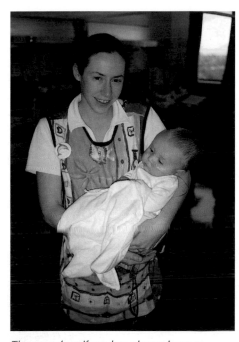

The nurse's uniform has always been a symbol of status, regardless of the impracticality of uniforms for work tasks and their potential to create a barrier between patients and nurses. In children's nursing, the traditional nurse's uniform has been replaced by more practical clothing. This senior grade nurse works in a London teaching hospital. (Photo: Deborah Ratnavel)

Not all children's nurses have abandoned the 'high status' uniform. (Photo: Mike Levers)

Efficiency and equity

At a most fundamental level, the key dilemma to be explored is the extent to which *efficiency* can be balanced with *equity* or 'fairness', and the ways in which these goals can be reconciled. How can efficiency balance costs and quality of health care and how can they be reconciled? Would the issues of quality of life and of death be the same as for the manufacture of, for example, video recorders? Similarly, the notion of efficiency might not be easily reconciled with considerations of equity (the equity–efficiency trade-off was discussed in Chapter 2). Perhaps more generally, the public might look to the government to act as a model employer in balancing equitable considerations with those of efficiency in its treatment of its own workers, rather than running the risk of exploiting them because few equivalent jobs exist in the private sector.

This raises the questions of how the differing concerns of employers, workers and the public can be settled and how important is the relative power of these groups in mediating outcomes? The general dilemma of equity and efficiency is often expressed through specific and tangible dilemmas concerning the processes through which pay should be determined. The levels at which pay outcomes should be set, for a large and complex workforce, as well as who is to do what in terms of the **grademix** (appropriate mix of grades) and what 'productivity', or workload, ideally should be are all parts of this dilemma.

This chapter discusses how concerns with a narrow definition of efficiency and a focus on perennial costs have frequently threatened to overwhelm notions of equity and quality, and have produced, in practice, an NHS workforce which is organised in a hierarchy divided by class, gender and ethnicity. Private-sector management techniques, which have long been employed in the NHS, are the subject both of conflict within a highly unionised workforce and of electoral concern. At the same time, health workers and the public have often been standard-bearers for the importance of quality.

'Nursing staff' and 'nurses' are generic terms used throughout this chapter as shorthand for nurses, midwives and health visitors. However, it should be noted that midwives and health visitors have a distinctly different training and role, although they often share a common foundation training programme.

5.2   Controlling the paybill: balancing efficiency and equity

The general dilemma of achieving a balance between efficiency and equity in the NHS comes into sharp focus when considering the specifics of health-service employer and worker strategies and objectives around pay, grademix, and productivity.

One key resource issue for employers in a highly labour-intensive sector like the NHS is how to control the paybill, where this is the main item in revenue expenditure. Table 5.1 presents a breakdown of NHS Trust and Health Authority expenditure over a five-year period from 1994 to 1998.

Table 5.1   Analysis of Health Authority and NHS Trust expenditure in England, 1994–98 (year-end 31 March).

| | £millions | | | | |
	1994	1995	1996	1997	1998
salaries and wages	13 913	14 303	14 961	15 580	16 099
supplies and services:					
clinical	2053	2219	2410	2599	2849
general	464	482	507	523	634
establishment	637	670	703	700	869
transport and moveable plant	115	121	132	141	not available
premises and fixed plant	1455	1576	1600	1592	1560
miscellaneous expenditure	1470	1391	1510	1069	1145
capital	1558	1107	1157	1069	1065
purchase of health care from non-NHS bodies	325	586	731	726	1108
external contract staff	106	118	178	129	not available
total revenue expenditure	**22 096**	**22 573**	**23 890**	**24 128**	**25 329**

Source: Department of Health website (www.doh.gov.uk/public/stats.3htm Tbl E3, accessed on 26 July 2001).

● According to Table 5.1, what is the largest single item in the expenditure?

■ Around 65 per cent of revenue expenditure in the NHS (over £16 billion in 1998) goes directly on salaries and wages, a figure which rises when indirect labour is also included (for example, contracted-out labour or other labour services provided by the private sector).

Government and managers concerned with managing the cost of the NHS are therefore necessarily concerned primarily with restraining labour cost.

● Suggest two ways in which staff payment could be reduced.

■ Two key ways of reducing payment are to reduce salaries and to increase productivity so that fewer staff are needed do the same work.

The highest part of the salary bill for the NHS is that of nursing staff and, for this reason, they are an important focus of this chapter.

5.2.1 Using divisions of labour to control costs

At the most direct level, government and managers may attempt to influence pay determination systems and restrain pay outcomes. A more subtle way of restraining the paybill, however, is the manipulation of the divisions of health-care labour. In its simplest form, this involves the substitution of cheaper for more expensive labour: thus through **labour substitution**, nurses may be substituted for doctors, or non-registered nursing staff or ancillary staff may be substituted for registered nurses. This could be effected through a reallocation of tasks with associated changes in training, or a simple redefinition of grade. Finally, employers may try to restrain labour costs by increasing productivity (or workload) in terms of output-per-worker, and putting a limit on the numbers employed. Thus, the attempt might be made to make people work harder, or for longer hours, or to exert more control over the way in which they work. However, each of these employer strategies, which turn on a narrow definition of efficiency focused on cost, might come into conflict with worker (and public) objectives on equity and quality.

Maintaining the balance between pay levels on the one hand and recruitment and retention on the other has been a dilemma throughout the history of formal health care. Similarly, grademix changes may also be deeply resisted by unions and professional associations, who are concerned both about the loss of professional jobs and about increases in workload and responsibility without fully corresponding increases in pay and status. Finally, there are limits to the amount and intensity of work people can perform before their own health or the quality of work performed is impaired — in a health-care setting this can have dangerous consequences. Once again, workers' professional unions and associations might, in particular, resist attempts to control the way that they work, particularly where this is seen to contradict their own concepts of safety and good practice.

The next section illustrates the ways in which competing strategies around the central dilemmas of pay and grademix have worked historically to form the modern NHS workforce. The dilemma of productivity in its modern context is discussed again in Section 5.5.

5.3 The historical roots of the division of health-care labour

An important part of understanding the modern division of health-care labour, and associated dilemmas, lies in the historical roots of this division in both the wider socio-economic system, and in the strategies pursued by employers and workers' representative organisations, mediated by public concern.

5.3.1 Early division of labour, worker associations and unions

The medical sociologists Margaret Stacey (1991) and Lesley Doyal with Imogen Pennell (1979) provide an important historical overview of the formalisation of health care, and the division of labour which subsequently emerged. They show that gender and class divisions in the wider economy and society were deeply influential. Prior to the eighteenth century, most health care was performed by women in the domestic domain, in households organised around the patriarchal family — a domestic group in which the husband/father had power and authority. Women were excluded from the outset from the London College of Physicians and, with the growth and formalisation of publicly provided health care in the eighteenth century, continued to be largely excluded from emergent medical roles whilst still providing health care at home. As Margaret Stacey states:

> ... the scene was laid in the arenas of public health and curative medicine, in both home and hospital, for the development and triumph of biomedicine in the nineteenth century as a male-dominated and class-based profession. (Stacey, 1991, p. 59)

● There are not only divisions between professions but also within professions. Suggest what divisions in nursing evolved as a result of the NHS reforms of the 1970s.

■ With the *Salmon reforms*, nurse leaders were taken away from bedside nursing. Domestic tasks became increasingly separated from nursing, and nursing auxiliaries carried out some of the less technical aspects of care.[1]

With women excluded from the emerging medical professions, nursing and ancillary roles were in turn divided internally on the basis of class and gender distinctions, which largely reflected the class-based provision of health care itself and wider gender stereotypes and constraints. Health care in Britain was built on a Victorian system of Poor Law workhouses and asylums in which the working poor, paupers and their aged relatives were treated, and voluntary hospitals, where the middle classes were treated alongside some of the 'better-off' working class or sponsored poor. The wealthy however were treated privately. Workhouse facilities and asylums were staffed mainly and respectively by working-class women and men. The voluntary sector offered more opportunity for middle-class women to enter nursing, supported by a greater number of untrained working-class women.

In the latter part of the nineteenth century, upper- and middle-class women attempted to redefine nursing into a respectable occupation for themselves and for some working-class women. Yet, Brian Abel-Smith (1960) argues in his classic history that the model of nursing that emerged was deeply patriarchal, hierarchical

[1] The *Salmon Report* of 1966 and the increase in employment of nursing auxiliaries is discussed in *Caring for Health: History and Diversity* (Open University Press, 3rd edn, 2001), Ch. 6.

and class conscious. Moreover, as Margaret Stacey has written, the ethos was one that stressed 'vocation, selflessness and dedication' (Stacey, 1991, p. 109). Nurses continued to be the handmaidens of doctors, despite increasing professionalisation.

Representation of health workers

The professional associations and trade unions that began to form by the early twentieth century were divided along lines which clearly reflected these divisions within health-care labour. Doctors and dentists were already represented (respectively) by the British Medical Association (BMA, established 1832) and British Dental Association (BDA, established 1880), both among the earliest professional associations. The **professions allied to medicine** (PAMs), for example, radiographers, physiotherapists and speech therapists, also established their own associations from the late nineteenth century onwards. Within nursing, a wide variety of associations arose, located mainly in the upper echelons of the voluntary sector and sharing a common goal of professionalism and *closure* for the nursing profession. This meant that they were concerned, via national standards of training and examination, to 'draw a firm line between those who were fitted to practice as nurses and those who were not' (Abel-Smith, 1960, p. 61). The College of Nursing founded in 1916, and later to become the Royal College of Nursing (RCN), emerged as the dominant association following formal registration of nurses in 1919 by Act of Parliament. However, student nurses were not admitted prior to 1926, nor male nurses until 1960. Unqualified nurses were excluded by definition.

Partly in reaction to the conservatism and exclusive nature of the professional associations, trade unions were also formed which represented in particular the interests of working-class workers lower down the health hierarchy, or those excluded by the professional associations. Early trade unions represented Poor Law and asylum workers, and recruited amongst administrative and clerical, ancillary and nursing grades. The associations were more concerned with achieving professional closure, and the pay and conditions of most health workers remained generally poor. The unions therefore sought to win status by campaigning for material improvements and trying to recruit qualified staff, a point we return to in Section 5.6.2.

5.3.2 Employer strategies

From the outset, state and employer strategies tended to foster and exploit divisions, particularly within nursing, both through manipulation of pay systems and outcomes, and through labour substitution.

Prior to the formation of the NHS, the health-care system itself, and the largely local pay systems associated with it, had become disorganised and fragmented. Within the key area of nursing, employers tended to foster the associations as a bulwark against trade unionism, with most nurses 'outside the scope of collective bargaining' (Clegg and Chester, 1957, p. 4) altogether. The resultant poor pay-outcomes became associated with endemic shortages and bad industrial relations.

Public concern tended to crystallise around *nursing shortages* and by the advent of World War II, this combined with wider labour movement pressure for a fundamental overhaul of the pay system. However, national pay arrangements made during the war were again biased in favour of the nursing associations, which then carried forward into the new centralised national collective-bargaining system, namely the Whitley general and functional councils, with the establishment of the NHS in 1948. Preference was given to more conservative associations in successive changes to pay determination systems, which tended to hold back improvements in pay and conditions. This bias was then compounded by government's *de facto* use of cash limits and pay restraint from the outset, and nursing shortages caused by poor pay-outcomes have continued throughout the post-World War II era (Thornley, 1996a).

Labour substitution as part of employer policy has also been visible throughout the twentieth century, particularly in nursing where the delineation and ownership of nursing skills remained a contested terrain. Prior to World War II, employers increasingly used unqualified nurses on the wards. Labour substitution practices were then continued in the new NHS, with the introduction of Enrolled Nurses (ENs) in 1943, and the formal recognition and expansion of the Nursing Auxiliary (NA) role in 1955. Both grades drew on married women, part-timers, the less educationally advantaged and more working class, and on ex-colonial and commonwealth recruitment. These strategies thus acted to reinforce gender, class, and ethnic divisions.

Many 'unqualified' people continued to engage in duties that could be defined as nursing, and many nurses in duties that could be defined as auxiliary.

5.3.3 Modern contradictions of the system (1979–90)

The paradox of employer strategies on pay restraint and labour substitution is that they gave rise to a cycle in which relatively poor pay, shortages and increases in workers at the lower end of the hierarchy all contributed to rising discontent, a growth in trade union membership, and a more militant approach by health-service workers. This was accompanied by ever-present public concern about health-care provision, expressed not least through electoral influence.

● Suggest some of the short- and long-term consequences of keeping the salary of nurses as low as possible.

■ In the short term, recruitment and retention problems may be experienced; in the longer term, nurses might leave the profession altogether because they find low pay inequitable. Alternatively, low pay may cause low morale and/or industrial conflict. Either outcome is likely to create public concern and ultimately affect patient care.

The RCN adopted trade union status in 1977 and membership of the TUC-affiliated unions greatly expanded. Industrial unrest over government-imposed wage restraint erupted in the early 1980s, with around three million working days lost in the NHS dispute of 1981–82 (*Hansard*, 18 January 1983). Employer responses have followed the historical focus on pay and grademix outlined above. First, a Review Body for Nurses, Midwives, Health Visitors and PAMs was established in 1983; it is an independent body whose unpaid members are appointed by the Prime Minister to advise on the remuneration of NHS staff in Great Britain. Secondly, there have been fresh attempts at labour substitution (the so-called 'skillmix' exercises) culminating in the introduction in 1990 of a new grade of health worker, the Health Care Assistant (or HCA). Here, strategies on pay restraint and on labour substitution coalesce.

Both low pay and substitution strategies were highly important in the 1990s (along with a variety of other techniques more commonly associated with the private sector) and are discussed in more detail in Section 5.6. However, at this stage, we provide a snapshot of the modern NHS workforce to give a more detailed context for the key issues at the turn of the twenty-first century.

5.4 The modern NHS division of labour

Numbers of occupational groups in health care

A snapshot of health-service staff in Great Britain is provided in Table 5.2, which covers changes in employment numbers from 1981 to 1998. It can be seen that nurses, midwives and health visitors still form the largest single occupational group in direct-care provision.

Table 5.2   Health Service staff in Great Britain, 1981–98.[a]

	Thousands				
	1981	**1986**	**1991**	**1994**	**1998**
NHS Hospital and Community Health Service (HCHS) staff					
medical and dental staff	48	51	56	60	70
nursing, midwifery and health visitors	457	472	470	426	407
other non-medical staff	473	436	429	432	448
total HCHS staff	**978**	**959**	**955**	**918**	**927**
Family Health Services (FHS) staff					
general medical practitioners	27	29	31	32	35
general dental practitioners	15	17	18	19	20
total FHS staff	**42**	**46**	**49**	**51**	**55**
ALL HEALTH-CARE STAFF	**1 020**	**1 005**	**1 004**	**969**	**982**

Source: *Social Trends – 30*, Office of National Statistics, The Stationery Office, London, 2000, Table 8.13, p. 139.

[a] Adapted from the HCHS non-medical workforce census; this is a large statistical exercise collecting over 800 000 records from about 500 contributors. Its aim is to provide *estimates* of the number of staff employed by the HCHS in order to allow comparisons to be made over time, and act as a framework for more detailed analysis. Hence totals given are not necessarily exactly the sum of the numbers in the groups of staff.

Using the data in Table 5.2, answer the following questions.

● What are the main changes in NHS Hospital and Community Health Services (HCHS) staff from 1981 to 1998?

■ Despite the rise in medical and dental staff (from 48 000 to 70 000), there has been an overall decline in numbers of HCHS staff employed. This means that the decline in nursing and other non-medical staff is comparatively more acute.

● What percentage of the overall health-care workforce did general medical and dental practitioners (i.e. Family Services) account for in 1998?

■ Just under six per cent.

Despite the rise in the number of doctors, demand for their services actually exceeds the numbers employed nationally, locally or by specialty. For example, England has one of the lowest numbers of physicians per head of population of all the member countries of the Organisation for Economic Cooperation and Development.

A slightly more detailed breakdown for HCHS staff for England is provided in Table 5.3 (*overleaf*), which shows changes in the ten years from 1988 to 1998. It should be noted, however, that the method of accounting for staff changed in 1995 and this has caused problems in extrapolating and interpreting longer-term trends.

Table 5.3 NHS Hospital and Community Health Services: directly employed staff by main staff groups in England at 30 September, 1988–98. (See the footnote to Table 5.2)

	Full-time equivalent (thousands)						
	1988	1993	1994	1995	1996	1997	1998
all direct care staff				497.3	507.9	508.3	517.3
nursing, midwifery and health visiting				330.4	332.7	330.6	332.2
of which:							
qualified staff				246.8	248.1	246.0	247.2
medical and dental	42.8	48.7	49.4	52.6	54.2	57.1	58.7
other direct care staff				111.6	118.5	120.6	126.4
all management and support staff				260.9	255.9	249.7	248.6
administration and estates staff				168.7	167.4	167.0	167.7
other management and support staff				92.2	88.4	82.8	80.9
all directly employed staff	**787.2**	**769.1**	**758.5**	**755.6**	**761.3**	**758.1**	**765.9**

Source: Department of Health (1999) *Statistical Bulletin 1999/12*, The Stationary Office, London; www.doh.gov.uk.

● What is the general trend in numbers of all directly employed staff?

■ Once again, a decline is easily visible.

● What percentage do all management and support staff account for, and what has been the trend in numbers since 1995?

■ Around 32 per cent, with numbers declining from 1995. (However, the way in which the staff categories are put together hides a rise in administrative and management staff; see Section 5.4.1).

● What is the trend in numbers of 'qualified' nursing staff and 'other direct care staff' from 1995 to 1998?

■ The numbers of 'qualified' nursing staff have remained broadly static, while numbers of other direct care staff have risen.

While Tables 5.2 and 5.3 provide a broad overview of NHS staff trends, it is necessary to understand in more detail what underlies them.

5.4.1 Occupations and trends

Table 5.4 shows the percentage of care staff working in different occupational categories within the NHS as defined by the Department of Health and provides a more detailed picture of how the categories are comprised. While some of the workers listed under 'HCAs and support staff' correspond in part to a previous 'ancillary' category, which encompassed catering, cleaning and portering, many are engaged in nursing duties. This is a complex category, and the official statistics are problematic (see below). A more disaggregate breakdown is of course possible. Around three-quarters of nurses, midwives and health visitors are defined as qualified staff, and a quarter are nursing auxiliaries. Table 5.4 shows the settings in which

Table 5.4 Breakdown of occupational categories within the NHS in England in 2000. (See the footnote to Table 5.2.)

Occupational category	Percentage
Medical and dental staff	8
Nurses, midwives and health visitors	44
of which:	
acute, elderly and general area of nursing	52
psychiatry (including community)	16
learning difficulties	7
community services	12
maternity services	8
paediatric nursing	5
HCAs and support staff	11
Scientific, therapeutic and technical staff	14
which include the main categories of	
pathology staff	19
physiotherapy staff	14
occupational therapy staff	12
radiography staff	11
pharmacy staff	9
other groups	35
Administrative and estates staff	22
of which:	
senior managers	5
other administrative managers	9
clerical and administrative staff	79
maintenance and works staff	7
Ambulance and other staff	2

Table compiled by the U205 course team from data in Department of Health (2000) *Statistical Bulletin 2000/11*, The Stationery Office, London; www.doh.gov.uk.

they work, and not surprisingly over half of them work in the acute, elderly and general area of nursing. Community midwives, district nurses and health visitors are all by definition qualified staff, and constitute around 12 per cent of the whole nursing workforce. In addition to these HCHS staff, just over 10 600 practice nurses work in General and Personal Medical Services.

The other major categories can be broken down in a similar way. For example, Table 5.4 also shows some of the sub-categories of 'scientific, therapeutic and technical staff', and 'administrative and estates staff'.

Longer-term trends

When categories of staff are broken down into their constituent parts, the statistics raise different concerns. For example, the longer-term trends (1989–99) show an overall fall in nursing staff with a stagnation in 'qualified' nursing staff numbers and an increase of 14 per cent in the number of 'unqualified' staff including HCAs (Department of Health, 2000d). At the same time there has been an increase of one-third over the ten-year period in the number of scientific, professional and technical staff. The reasons for the increase in technical staff is discussed in Chapter 7 of this book.

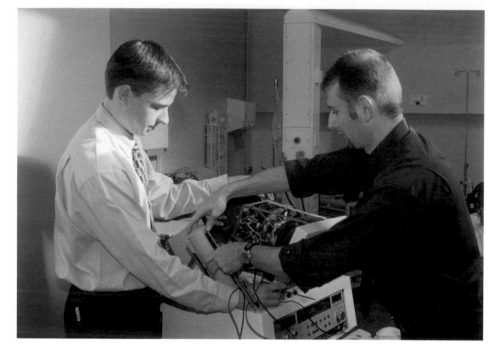

The increasing use of medical technology has resulted in a rise in the number of staff needed to support its application and use. Here, hospital technicians are repairing a piece of essential equipment. (Photo: Mike Levers)

Hospitals and community-care settings are becoming increasingly dependent upon technical support. Ancillary/support staff fell by 44 per cent over the period 1989–99, with similar reductions in maintenance and works staff, largely as a result of the contracting-out of support services. You may remember from Chapter 3 that there has been an increase in administrative staff (including managers), who increased by 39 per cent from 1989 to 1999. It is interesting to note that nursing staff numbers in the *private* hospitals, homes and clinics sector continued to increase in the late 1990s.

5.4.2 Class, gender and ethnicity

In line with historical development, Lesley Doyal and Imogen Pennell argued (1979) that the NHS hierarchy clearly reflected the wider class system, in terms of the privileges enjoyed by particular social groups with respect to pay, status and power, and the division of labour in society.

Subsequently, while noting problems with defining class, Margaret Stacey argued that:

> Some things are fairly clear however. No part of the medical profession, despite the variation in its power, remuneration and life-style, could be called proletarian in any strict sense. On the other hand, ancillary workers (porters, cleaners and other manual workers) by virtue of their terms and conditions of work, their remuneration, and their place in the division of labour are undoubtedly proletarian. There is evidence ... that nurses are

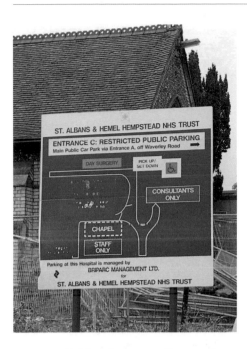

Hospital consultants continue to enjoy privileges that other professional groups do not. This sign illustrates a continuity of uncontested privilege, that of reserved parking spaces. (Photo: Mike Levers)

divided between those who are members of the proletariat ... and (those) who could definitely be called middle class on account also of their working situations. (Stacey, 1991, p. 189)

'Consultant nurses' or 'super nurses' describe a top clinical grade for nurses who spend a minimum of 50 per cent of their time working directly with patients, as well as contributing to the development of professional practice, research and education.

● What is the likely consequence of the introduction of nurse graduates and consultant nurses alongside an increase in non-registered nursing workforce?

■ The introduction of these nurses may indicate some tendency towards a widening of class differences *within* occupations as opposed to a breaking down of class barriers *between* occupations.

Around 80 per cent of the HCHS workforce is female (Department of Health, 2000e). Despite this, women are under-represented at the top of the hierarchy and over-represented in the lower echelons. For example, at the end of the twentieth century, women formed the overwhelming majority of the clerical and administrative workforce, but only half of administrative managers; in the mid-1990s, over 80 per cent of Trust Chief Executives were male (IDS, 1996). Moreover, despite an increase in the total number of female hospital medical staff of 73 per cent between 1989 and 1999, this still meant only a third of medical staff were female and they are again under-represented in the higher grades and certain specialities; for example, females only formed 5 per cent of surgical consultants in 1999 (Department of Health, 2000e). Similarly, despite the fact that nearly all the increase in GP numbers between 1989 and 1999 occurred amongst women, only 34 per cent of GPs are female (Department of Health, 2000d).

The great majority of HCAs and support staff are also female. Nursing, which has a workforce at just under 90 per cent female, represents the classic case of women's work, with evidence of both **horizontal** and **vertical segregation** (women being disproportionately employed in certain specialisms and in the lower parts of the grade hierarchy).

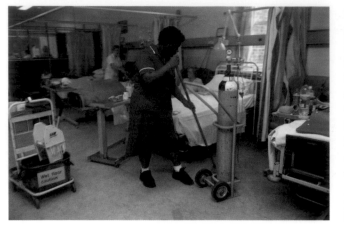

Women from black and ethnic minority groups are over-represented among hospital domestic staff. (Photo: John Harris/Report Digital)

Part-time work is also strongly associated with gender and tends to be more prevalent at lower levels of the hierarchy (for example, fluctuating at around 40 per cent in nursing). This latter feature, of course, raises important questions about division of domestic responsibilities and the need for 'family-friendly policies' at work. More generally, doubts have been raised about how a balance between work and personal lives can be achieved in practice for NHS staff as a whole, when one in six are also informal carers.

Finally, around 6 per cent of the HCHS workforce is from ethnic minority groups, with these groups over-represented in the lower-paid occupations of nursing, where the highest numbers are to be found amongst nursing auxiliaries and health-care assistant/support workers. One exception to this general rule is the relatively high representation of ethnic minorities (particularly of Asian origin) amongst medical staff, for whom there is a history of overseas recruitment. Nonetheless, even here, such doctors are under-represented in the most senior grades of consultant.

5.4.3   Trade union and professional representation

As argued previously, forms of worker representation have tended to reflect social divisions in class and gender, and employer/worker strategies. Despite the fact that the NHS workforce as a whole is one of the most highly unionised in the country, each profession, semi-profession or occupational group tends to have its own association or union, and these divisions, exacerbated by a degree of competition between organisations, may have enabled employers to 'divide and rule'.

However, some important changes have occurred in recent years. Three trade unions merged in 1993 to form the largest union in the country, UNISON. This union now represents workers across the health hierarchy, has just under half the NHS workforce in membership, and shares representation of nurses with the second largest union in the NHS, the Royal College of Nursing (RCN). Secondly, some of the 'professional' associations and unions have shown a tendency to become more 'unionate' in behaviour, in the sense of deploying tactics more traditionally associated with trade unions: one expression of this, as Frank Burchill (a professor of industrial relations) and Alice Casey (a director of human resources in a large NHS Trust), have put it, is a movement, 'towards increased, and more devolved, use of the method of collective bargaining' (Burchill and Casey, 1996, p. 54). While the overall picture can still be interpreted as a divided one, and there are still important differences, these changes may prove very significant.

5.4.4   Current pay systems and rates

The divisions discussed above are, of course, reflected both in pay systems and rates (see Section 5.3.3). The pay hierarchy as a whole generally reflects that in wider society. Research from the mid-to-late 1990s found that NHS Trust Chief Executives earned just under four times a registered nurse's average gross salary, while hospital doctors earned just over two-and-a-half times this latter amount (Thornley, 1996b, 1998a).

● From your reading of Chapter 3, recall the range of salary paid to hospital managers and explain why this is significant in this context.

■ The salary for managers in the NHS in 2000 ranged from just over £16 000 to almost £100 000 and it could be argued, therefore, that pay divisions within this professional group are wider than those within nursing.

Despite the differences within professional groups, differences between those at the top of the hierarchy and people at the 'sharp end' remain the main focus of discontent. For example, average Chief Executives' pay was reported as at least £80 000, while nursing auxiliaries received an average gross salary of around £11 000 (ONS, 1999). This begs the question of whether or not a Chief Executive is worth seven times more than a non-registered nurse.

Female nurses still earn less on average than male nurses (reflecting the greater propensity of male nurses to rise in the hierarchy), and differentials between registered and non-registered nurses have been widening. The same research also showed that around three-quarters of the nursing workforce are found in grades A to E (ranging from £7 955 to £17 830 in 1999 (Review Body for Nursing Staff, 2000) while around one-third suffer low basic pay, as defined by the Council of Europe decency threshold definitions. The use of HCAs has introduced a growing problem of low pay as their rates undercut existing Whitley rates: the average basic salary for an HCA in the late 1990s was just under £9 000. Low pay is also prevalent in administrative, clerical and ancillary grades. At the time of writing, in July 2001, UNISON is playing a leading role by backing 'Europe's largest equal pay case … forcing the Department of Health into an emergency review of pay structures to avoid a total compensation bill for female staff that could reach 15 billion pounds.' (*Observer*, 15 July 2001, p. 2). Although the industrial tribunal case is still going on, this has set an important marker for the future.

5.5 Current dilemmas and controversies

In this and the next concluding section, the focus is on the main dilemmas of the 1990s in nursing and what are likely to be the preoccupations of the next decade. It will be clear to you that 'nothing is new' in that historical dilemmas seem to be reflected, and sometimes reinforced, in modern trends.

The effects of cheap labour

At this point, you might like to pause and consider some of the key issues arising from the historical roots and modern form of the NHS division of labour. Taking expenditure as a proportion of Gross Domestic Product (GDP), the NHS represents one of the cheapest forms of health-service provision in advanced industrial economies.

● From the strategies outlined in Section 5.4, what dilemmas arise from attempts to make the NHS more cost-effective?

■ The chief dilemma is that apparent signs of efficiency may be achieved at the expense of equity where pay is such a large component of cost, and changes may exacerbate class and gender divisions within and between occupational groups, as well as contributing to a drift towards low pay. This in turn may cause recruitment and retention problems — an efficiency issue.

Clearly, some might argue that the comparative 'cheapness' of the NHS represents a more general sign of underfunding, underprovision and underpayment of health-service workers.

Locally determined pay

Employer strategies in the 1990s have focused on pay systems and substitution. With respect to pay systems, the 1990 NHS and Community Care Act, introduced by the Conservative government, not only established the notion of NHS Trusts but also the notion of *locally determined pay*, which would depart from established national Whitley rates. Research into the local pay experiment showed this to be unworkable (Thornley, 1998b). However, while the Conservative government changed its mind just prior to the 1997 general election, remnants of local pay determination remain for some NHS workers — in particular, for HCAs. Moreover, the Labour government which succeeded to power in 1997, quickly engaged in discussions on a new pay system to be based on national pay spines with local flexibilities.

It would seem that employers may be no closer to an 'ideal' pay system now than they have been in the past. The potentially fragmented and decentralised (or even privatised) systems of the future may prove highly problematic, and have the potential to exacerbate existing pay inequalities.

Substitution and grademix

With respect to substitution and grademix, the 1990 NHS and Community Care Act also introduced the 'new' grade of HCA. The substitution of nurses for doctors has been a crucial part of the general reduction in junior doctors' hours, and HCAs in particular have been used to substitute not only for registered nursing staff, but also for other occupations further up the hierarchy (as we describe in Section 5.6). Employer strategy has to a large extent focused on the division of labour in health care, with an emphasis on reassigning tasks across occupational categories, while developing grades that will carry out this work without fully achieving corresponding recognition or status. For example, in April 2000, the Secretary of State for Health expressed the wish to see health professions:

> ... working more flexibly, breaking down traditional barriers and demarcations ....We want to see an NHS in which staff work more flexibly, in which they are not confined by an outdated view of what is appropriate for particular professions to do and where they use the full range of their skills for the benefit of patients ....This means changes to the way in which staff are educated, trained, regulated and used by the NHS. (Department of Health, 2000f)

At the same time, there is little evidence to date that staff 'flexibility' will be fully compensated for in pay terms, and there is a continuing problem of low and unequal pay throughout the NHS, with associated labour shortages. Because of the crisis in recruitment and retention, extra resources have been promised for the NHS to bring funding closer to European levels over time, including a commitment to recruiting thousands of extra nurses. However, it remains unclear whether current pay rates will be sufficient to support this policy, and whether modest improvements in registered nurses' pay made in the late 1990s will be adequate to attract and retain staff. The new (and very numerically limited) grade of 'nurse consultants' has already attracted criticism for the restricted use of possible pay rates. Furthermore, a policy designed to have an incentive effect could fail if there are not sufficient posts available or they are not properly resourced.

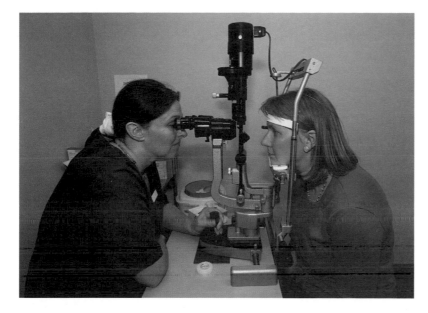

A nurse consultant uses a slit-lamp to check a patient's eye for 'foreign bodies'. This procedure may previously have been undertaken only by a member of the medical staff. (Photo: John Callan, Shout)

● What are the potential effects of creating more nurse consultant posts on current pay rates?

■ The posts could exacerbate divisions and pay differentials between registered and non-registered nurses, while doing little to close the gap between the average pay of, for example, doctors and nurses, or managers and nurses.

Controlling production, controlling labour

It is also possible to detect important recent developments in attempting to increase productivity through increased control of labour. Arguably, such increases may follow on more from the impact of tight central financial controls on employment, rather than from local initiatives. What is not contentious is the workload increase itself — as the Review Body for nurses notes:

> Whilst output from the NHS has risen, the total nursing workforce has remained static, supporting the view that both productivity and workload have increased. (Review Body for Nursing Staff, 2000, p. 24)

These increases in workload raise questions about their impact on absenteeism and job satisfaction. Another interesting development concerns changes in shift systems, including **internal rotation** (a system of working varying numbers of night and day shifts each month), rather than individual fixed-day/night systems. These rotas also appear to be a source of conflict, not least because of their adverse effect on the ability of staff on low incomes to supplement their earnings by attracting enhanced payments.

In sum, recent debates make clear that low pay and staff shortages remain contentious issues. One of the key features of the 'local pay experiment' was the extent to which professional associations and trade unions achieved a relative degree of unity in resisting what they perceived to be an unfair and deleterious change (Thornley, 1998b). The best way to advance health workers' interests remains a key issue for the variety of associations and unions. There remain important tensions between the aspirations of trade unions and professional associations organised around the central principle of closure, and those like UNISON organised around the central principle of achieving material improvements for all staff. The evidence suggests that the 'local pay experiment' also produced some shifts in membership towards UNISON.

A very important feature of this debate concerns appropriate levels of education, training, and career mobility, a set of issues considered next.

5.6   Case study: health-care assistants and nursing auxiliaries

In recent years, there has been a quiet revolution in the profile of the non-registered care-giving workforce in the NHS, and our understanding of these workers. The traditional grade of Nursing Auxiliary (NA) was rapidly expanded after achieving formal recognition in 1955. Throughout the 1980s it accounted for around one-quarter of the total nursing workforce. Yet the grade itself and the people who constitute it received negligible attention. Jane Salvage noted that NAs 'are a neglected group of people', with 'virtually no serious, extended discussion of the role auxiliaries play in caring for patients, despite its importance' (Salvage, 1985). Both Salvage and Celia Davies (Professor of Nursing at the Open University) (Davies, 1995) pointed to the fact that much direct care is carried out by NAs.

The lack of evidence in this area became significant when the HCA was introduced in 1990, and appeared to mark a new era of labour substitution. The 'new' grade was to have pay locally determined, in marked contrast to NAs whose pay was determined nationally by the nurses' Review Body within the Whitley system. Paradoxically, the impetus for this change arose in the mid-1980s, with a drive from the 'professionalising' elements in nursing for changes in nurse education to a more academic system. This impetus was realised in the set of initiatives which became known as Project 2000.

An associated aim for the professionalisers was that assistants to nurses should no longer have 'nurse' in the title so that the role of assistants would be fully distinguished from that of registered nurses. The Conservative government of the time pushed ahead with proposals for National Vocational Qualifications (NVQ) certificates for the new grade, while also intensifying a series of initiatives around so-called 'skillmix' and 'reprofiling' of the nursing workforce.

The following case study focuses on the special case of HCAs and illustrates in a marked form the themes discussed above with respect to pay, grademix and productivity. It draws on analysis and findings from a series of independent national research reports by the author from 1997 to 1999 (Thornley, 1997, 1998c, 1999, commissioned by UNISON).

5.6.1   Empirical evidence on HCAs and NAs

Research revealed a lack of reliable or accurate official data on the numbers of NAs and HCAs employed in the NHS, as well as confusion in official accounts between the roles of HCAs and support workers (Thornley, 1998c). This confusion has been exacerbated by the fact that HCAs have been introduced locally under a wide variety of titles, and are also being used in support roles to PAMs.

The cost-effectiveness of labour substitution

Managers reported 'cost-effectiveness' as the main reason for introducing HCAs. In line with this, the research found that local pay and conditions for HCAs substantially undercut the already low national Whitley rates for NAs. However, there was a high degree of agreement between managers, HCAs and NAs on actual roles performed; crucially, and irrespective of title used for HCAs, both groups of worker engage widely in nursing duties, with the job titles of NA and HCA now used almost interchangeably in most Trusts.

A detailed comparison of the work content of NAs and HCAs has shown these to be almost identical, with some workers in both grades — sometimes substantial minorities — also engaging extensively in a wide variety of more 'technical and advanced' tasks. These latter include: liaising directly with, or assisting, doctors; being in charge of a shift; looking after students or newly qualified nurses and agency staff; performing cardiac massage in cases of cardiac arrest. In fact, a majority of both grades reported that they 'undertake the same or similar work as a registered nurse' sometimes or frequently, with over half reporting that 'little' or 'none' of their work is supervised. These findings provide clear evidence of labour substitution.

The gender division of labour

The characteristics of these workers were remarkably similar regardless of whether they were categorised under the NA or HCA occupational grade. Over four-fifths of both groups were female, with around two-fifths to a half working part-time; in each instance, the great majority were aged over 30, with around half aged over 40; each exhibited overwhelming evidence of both formal and informal caring experience prior to taking up their current role. Each also exhibited a striking length of service in NHS caring, with associated experiential learning, and each also tended to undertake a degree of 'self-teaching'. Well over half had caring responsibilities at home.

The status of care work

The research also revealed that, despite problems with provision of training by Trusts, NVQ attainment is gradually becoming an expectation for both HCAs and NAs: around one-third had NVQ certificates; many more were currently attempting an NVQ or would like to do so. For many this was not so much a matter of learning new skills as one of gaining the formal qualifications that gave accreditation for already existing competencies.

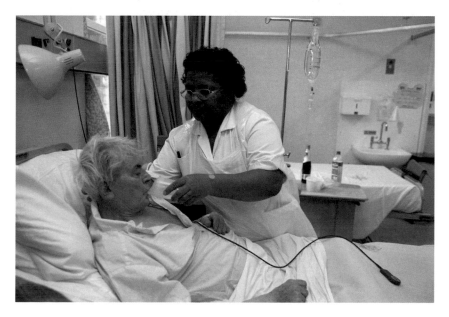

*A health-care assistant helps
an older patient to drink.
(Photo: John Harris, Report Digital)*

Open University students should now read the article entitled 'Professionalism and the conundrum of care', by Celia Davies in Davey, B., Gray, A. and Seale, C., *Health and Disease: A Reader* (Open University Press; 3rd edn 2001).

● What does Celia Davies see as the danger inherent in the new professionalism of nursing? How might this trend impact on NAs and HCAs?

■ She argues that nurses run the risk of losing the value of their caring role because caring carries a strong association with women's work. The nature of the 'soft' skills of nursing work conflicts with professionalising strategies in nursing which emphasise 'male, technical' skills. It would seem that HCAs and NAs are being undervalued on both counts.

This is consistent with the audiotape 'Who cares?', in which informal carers complained about the lack of acknowledgement of their role and status, despite society's and the health service professionals' obvious dependence upon their contribution to care. Part of their complaint related to the lack of value placed upon the 'caring role'.

5.6.2 Discussion and implications

The case of HCAs provides an apt illustration of the combined effects of a change in pay mechanism (from national to local), and of labour substitution, in driving down costs in the labour-intensive health-care system. Here, it can be seen that a new inequality in the health division of labour has been created, which builds on older divisions and a prior lack of recognition of the real work conducted by NAs. At the core of this issue is a failure to agree what the real content and boundaries of 'nursing' work should be. HCAs and NAs are undervalued both as doing women's work and as 'non-professionals'.

Excluding HCAs from the Royal College of Nursing

However, the story does not end there. In line with findings for registered nurses, both HCAs and NAs report stress problems and high intentions to leave, associated with having to work harder. Turnover is particularly high for HCAs. At the same time, both HCAs and NAs have relatively high union membership within UNISON, and improvements are being sought. Paradoxically, the RCN has until very recently resisted taking HCAs into membership:

> We are a trade union for professional nurses, not HCAs or other
> members allied to nursing. I do not believe it's in the interests of
> our organisation to admit these members. (Cowan, 2000, p. 5)

The Department of Health has acknowledged the importance of HCAs in the development of the NHS, and a review is also taking place on the potential for registration of HCAs.

Efficiency and equity

The case study of HCAs provides a modern example of historical tensions around the central issue of efficiency and equity. On a narrow definition of efficiency, a 'new' grade of worker was introduced, by-passing national pay determination procedures and lowering pay, with work that quickly intensified and expanded. However, issues of equity and of broader conceptions of efficiency were soon raised: the real skills and tasks of this largely female workforce, almost identical to that of an existing, more highly paid grade (NAs), have not received due recognition; the associated low pay and lack of status are leading in turn to stress, turnover and potential industrial-relations problems. At the same time, the chapter also illustrates the fundamental tensions over 'care work', with respect to how it is defined and organised, and with what recognition and reward. The modern dilemma for the nursing 'profession' itself has been summarised by Ann Bradshaw of the RCN Institute:

> Professional boundaries, and the competence needed for new roles, have become far less distinct than they were in the past. This has brought confusion and paradox to the modern nursing identity. For example, the UK government has commended the introduction of specialist nursing roles ... while consulting on the need to define common core competencies for nurse education, including those needed for personal care such as assisting with washing and eating ... urgent debate is needed about the current mutation of the nursing role and the increasing loss of its foundational place in the bedside delivery of 'total patient care'. (Bradshaw, 2000, p. 328).

Professional boundaries

Changes in the NHS and their impact upon the role of nurses has resulted in a blurring of the professional boundaries. A smaller health-care group, PAMS, have also suffered from an identity 'crisis' as a result of these changes. Open University students should now read the article entitled 'Professions Allied to Medicine: continuity and change in a complex workforce', by Lesley Doyal and Ailsa Cameron in Davey, B., Gray, A. and Seale, C., *Health and Disease: A Reader* (Open University Press; 3rd edn 2001).

● From the study findings described in the article, what particular difficulties associated with their new roles have PAMS experienced?

■ PAMS experienced difficulties as a result of their low population as a professional group, their lack of representation in decision-making arenas and poor understanding of their particular skills by other health-care workers.

● How does the clinical accountability of PAMS differ from that of nurses?

■ Unlike nurses who belong to one discipline, PAMS in the study were accountable to several different managers in different discipline areas.

● How able are PAMS to protect their professional status?

■ The study found a variety of influences across occupational groups. Radiographers were a comparatively strong professional group in contrast to occupational therapists, whose professional independence was more vulnerable because of their lack of a medical power base.

It is clear from the study by Doyal and Cameron that divisions of health-care labour exist within and between professional groups. As a comparatively small professional group, PAMS suffer from low visibility and lack of representation, which has resulted in some groups being easily deskilled and subsequently becoming expendable!

5.7   Conclusion and prospects

This chapter has explored the historical roots of both the division of labour and divided representation. Divisions by class, gender and ethnicity in the complex hierarchical division of NHS labour reflect and reinforce those in the broader society. The key dilemma of attaining efficiency together with equity has been discussed, and illustrated with particular respect to the associated dilemmas concerning pay, grademix and productivity for the registered and non-registered nursing workforce.

It is still unclear whether governments will pursue traditional strategies, or attempt a more egalitarian and open management of NHS labour and lend some substance to the notion of government as a 'model employer'. There have been elements of both strategies in recent policy moves. It is similarly rather early to tell whether the NHS unions and associations can provide a more united front and countervailing power balance in the future and what the role of UNISON will be.

Clearly, this approach might entail a fundamental revision of notions of 'professionalism' and 'closure' and a more egalitarian approach to training, recognition and reward for all. Health care remains a key issue for the electorate, who equally seem to understand that its quality and quantity crucially depend on adequate numbers of, and reward for, experienced, trained and dedicated staff. In this way, public concern continues to galvanise politicians into action.

Such public concern is reflected in *The NHS Plan* (Department of Health, 2000a). Combined with a commitment to increased spending, as discussed in Chapter 2, there are a wide raft of proposals, which include some key provisions on NHS staff: an increase in employment (9 500 more consultants and GPs, 20 000 more nurses and 6 500 extra other health professionals); new contracts for consultants and GPs; and changed roles and responsibilities for nurses, midwives, therapists and other NHS staff. (The latter provision involves changes in the treatment of HCAs and NAs, educational change and the development of 'modern matrons' and nurse consultants.)

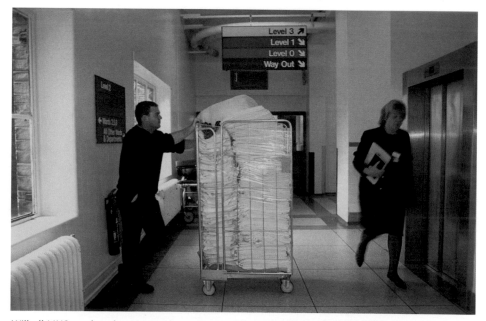

Will all NHS workers be prepared to unite in order to strengthen their bargaining position or are the divisions between groups too great? (Photo: United National Photographs)

The continuing centrality of division of labour issues is visible in the policy rhetoric of *The NHS Plan*, which challenges 'traditional professional boundaries', 'demarcations' and 'old hierarchical ways of working', promoting instead the language of 'flexible team working'. Taken alongside the structural proposals contained in the document for the NHS itself and proposals for an enhanced role for the private sector.

OBJECTIVES FOR CHAPTER 5

When you have studied this chapter, you should be able to:

5.1 Define and use, or recognise definitions and applications of, each of the terms printed in **bold** in the text.

5.2 Discuss the significance of the size and complexity of the NHS workforce for labour-cost control.

5.3 Comment on the main strategies available to government and managers who seek to contain workforce costs.

5.4 Describe the division of labour within the NHS workforce in terms of class, gender, ethnicity, occupation, pay and representation.

5.5 Discuss the extent to which nursing 'professionalisation' strategies can be considered successful in the light of history and current changes.

5.6 Describe the issues concerned with the professional status of PAMs, HCAs, and NAs.

QUESTIONS FOR CHAPTER 5

1 (*Objectives 5.2 and 5.3*)

What are the main cost-restraint strategies open to government and managers in relation to the NHS workforce? What problems do these strategies generate?

2 (*Objective 5.4*)

What factors contribute to an explanation of why doctors are still mostly male and nurses still overwhelmingly female?

3 (*Objective 5.5*)

'Boundaries between grades in nursing, and indeed boundaries between nursing and non-nursing duties seem impossible to set and nurses do whatever is necessary to ensure patient care.' (Celia Davies, 1995, p.7)

How successful have nursing 'professionalisation' strategies been?

4 (*Objective 5.6*)

Can HCAs or NAs be described as 'unskilled' or 'unqualified' staff? How can you account for the pay and conditions of HCAs being worse than those for NAs?

CHAPTER 6

Evaluating health care: dilemmas posed by research and evidence

Study notes for OU students

This chapter considers the more detailed dilemmas that arise from the process of evaluation. In Chapters 2 and 3, you were introduced to the dilemmas that result directly from economic processes and management. In this series, in *Studying Health and Disease* (Open University Press, colour-enhanced 2nd edn 2001), you were also introduced to randomised controlled trials (RCTs) and that knowledge is built upon here.

During your study of Section 6.5.1, you will be asked to read an article entitled 'Evidence-based medicine: what it is and what it isn't' by David L. Sackett and colleagues, and a reply from Alan Maynard published originally in the *British Medical Journal*, both of which appear in *Health and Disease: A Reader* (Open University Press, 3rd edn 2001).

This chapter is written by David Foxcroft, who is Professor of Health Care at Oxford Brookes University, and Carol Komaromy the book editor.

6.1   Evaluation as a process

The focus of this chapter's discussion is on the process of **health-care evaluation**, which involves assessing the impact of health interventions. This process encompasses four elements: clinical trials[1]; **health technology assessment**, the evaluation of the clinical effectiveness of new technologies; **clinical audit**, a cycle of setting standards for clinical care, monitoring performance and then implementing change to bring performance up to standard; and economic evaluation, as discussed in Chapter 2.

In order to set priorities, policy decision-makers in health care need to have good quality information about the effectiveness and efficiency of treatment interventions. Although drug trials have a long history, health-care providers were not consistently required to supply evidence of the effectiveness of their treatments until about the 1980s. Although evaluation is not a new process, more recently evidence has become the focus of attention within resource management.

A key problem in evaluation is that purchasers and providers have different objectives. Purchasers of health care need to know what interventions are efficacious and cost-effective and therefore provide the best value for money, whereas health-care professionals are required to provide care and treatment that, at best, promotes health, and at the least does not harm their patients. The evidence provided by evaluation has the potential to help to resolve this tension between the different objectives of purchasers and providers.

● What other evidence would you expect to be useful in facilitating and informing health-care decisions?

■ Not only is evidence about the cost-effectiveness and efficacy of treatments essential, but health-care systems, policy and procedures contribute to the process of decision-making and would ideally also be evaluated.

Evidence from evaluation provides useful information on which to base sound health-care decisions. However, the evaluation process is itself subject to dilemmas, and this chapter considers some of these in terms of what constitutes 'good' evidence, how evidence can be used most effectively and at what cost.

6.1.1   Making rational decisions

Within the medical model of health-care provision, a high value is placed upon scientific methods of evaluation to underpin 'rational' decision-making. In this context, 'rational' approaches are distinguished from the 'non-rational', such as following traditional routines in clinical decisions about treatment. However, the scientific focus has tended to undervalue or exclude evaluation of the social components of health, such as housing and education, in part because of the way that Western scientific medicine has evolved, but also because measuring the outcomes of social interventions is broad and complex. Taking a rational approach to medical research even within a tightly constrained research area is not without problems.

● Consider Figure 6.1, which depicts four steps of a rational decision-making process, and suggest why there might be problems at each step and what these problems are likely to be.

[1] Clinical trials, including randomised controlled trials (RCTs), are discussed in *Studying Health and Disease* (Open University Press, 2nd edn 1994; colour-enhanced 2nd edn 2001), Chapter 8.

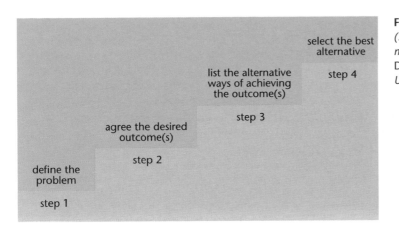

Figure 6.1 *Rational decision-making model. (Source: Based on a rational decision-making model in the Open University course, D208: Decision making in Britain, 1983, The Open University, Milton Keynes)*

■ Step 1: not everyone will agree about what is the problem. Step 2: the desired outcomes might differ according to different interests, and clinicians, patients and policymakers will not necessarily agree about the desired outcome. Step 3: listing the various ways of achieving the outcomes is a potentially endless procedure as there is a temptation to continue to gather evidence in the hope that it will solve the next stage. Step 4: this is based on the assumption that it is possible to establish the best way, but some options might be equally weighted and make the choice more difficult.

Not only is the decision-making process problematic, but the process of evaluation has inherent difficulties (as we discuss later in the chapter). Even when the decision about what action to take is based on evidence of the best option, the outcomes of the intervention also need to be evaluated. In the health-service context, this process is framed by the need to provide interventions that are efficient, efficacious and equitable as required by NHS care principles. Furthermore, it is the individual responsibility of NHS staff to base their practice on evidence. The clinical governance guidelines, as discussed in Chapter 3, form the framework through which quality and accountability are managed and require that:

> NHS organisations are accountable for improving the quality of their services and safeguarding high standards of care by creating an environment in which excellence in clinical care will flourish.
> (Roland and Baker, 1999, p. 3)

In evaluating health care, it is important to distinguish between **clinical products**, examples of which are drugs and surgical procedures, and **clinical processes**, that is the ways in which health care is organised, for example the pattern of visits from professionals such as community midwives, or the organisation of consultations between health professionals and patients. Evaluating the outcomes of health-care interventions necessarily involves attention to the interaction between products and processes, but they present different challenges for research.

● A palliative-care nurse visits a dying patient at home every day to administer pain-killing drugs via a syringe pump. Which aspects of this intervention would be most readily evaluated as to its effectiveness, and why? Which aspects would be hardest to evaluate?

■ The effectiveness of the clinical products (in this case the pain-killing drug and the syringe pump) could be most readily evaluated because their parameters (e.g. dosage, delivery rate, etc.) can be precisely controlled and compared with those of alternative products. The process of delivering palliative care is harder to evaluate because it could vary so much, e.g. in the pattern of visits, their duration, the procedures conducted each time, and because of the individuality of different nurse–patient interactions.

In summary, health-care evaluation, which is itself a process and not a single event, must take account of the complexity of health interventions in which some elements are intrinsically difficult to regulate. As a consequence of these difficulties, more attention has been focused on product evaluations than on the processes involved in health care.

6.1.2 Dilemmas in research and evidence

During the collection of evidence, which will take place over various time periods, decisions are needed on which parts should be prioritised, how evidence should be collected, how this evidence might be used, and how to evaluate clinical interventions where evidence is incomplete. Five important dilemmas arise from the generation and use of research evidence to support health-care decision-making.

First, is it more important to gather evidence for some health-care problems than for others? If so, what criteria can be used to determine priorities for evaluation, and which products, procedures or processes should take precedence? For example, a choice might have to be made between collecting evidence on the effectiveness of a new drug to treat heart disease or on the effectiveness of rehabilitation for people who have had a heart attack. Research commissioning by funding bodies, including the NHS, focuses upon national priorities, as in the case of coronary heart disease (as you will see in Chapter 8), but in publicly funded health-care systems a decision is often required between funding for one piece of research at the expense of another, equally worthy, research study.

Second, once decisions are made about priorities for evaluation, what sort of evaluation is appropriate? Certain types of evaluation method are costly and time-consuming, but are they always necessary? The '**gold standard**' of evidence in clinical research (which is discussed more fully in Section 6.3.1), is generally held to be randomised controlled trials (RCTs) systematically reviewed by experts, but is this always required, especially when it might mean that a number of other studies cannot be afforded? If gold standard research is not funded, then research findings can be more easily discounted, even to the extent that they may be regarded as worthless by some decision-makers. In many areas of clinical importance other types of study would be more appropriate than RCTs, but their outcomes may be undervalued.

Third, once evidence is available, how can it be used to support decisions on which health-care treatments and services should, and can, be afforded? Does using evidence as a basis for selecting services mean that areas with valid demands, but where there is little or no evidence, will come under increasing pressure from evidence-rich areas?

Fourth, what is the best way to translate evidence for approved treatments into clinical practice? One problem is that there is a trade-off between *locally* developed evidence-based guidelines, which are more likely to be adopted but run the risk of increasing the 'postcode lottery' of care, and national guidelines, which are more likely to be equitable but less likely to be implemented. Is it better to develop national guidelines and promote consistency, but risk a lower rate of implementation, or encourage local guideline development and promote uptake?

Finally, even though research evidence might indicate that certain treatments for particular illnesses are more effective than others, and these treatments are subsequently funded by the NHS, this does not mean that such treatments will always be preferred by patients. Individual choices lead to a further dilemma — should health policymakers work to maximise the uptake of an effective treatment, therefore increasing overall health gain within a population, but at the expense of individual patient choice?

In conclusion, the process of evaluation is based upon the privileged value afforded to data collected by scientific research and controlled trials. But even within this paradigm, the outcomes may still be contested and experts may continue to disagree about the value of the evidence.

6.1.3 What counts as evidence?

Good evidence on the benefits and drawbacks of an intervention ideally accumulates, to form a body of knowledge on what medical experts count as 'good' (or otherwise) for patients. This knowledge base is extremely important for health-care professionals, for if they are able to translate that knowledge into clinical practice, then it follows, in theory at least, that patients will benefit. This approach to interventions is called **evidence-based health care**. A more formal definition is provided by David Sackett, a clinical epidemiologist who collaborated in the creation of the Centre for Evidence-Based Medicine, and his colleagues, who state that:

> ... evidence-based health care aims to provide the means by which current best evidence from research can be judiciously and conscientiously applied in the prevention, detection and care of health disorders. (Sackett *et al.*, 1996, p. 72)

One alternative to evidence-based health care has been termed **eminence-based health care**. In this approach, the knowledge base on which clinical practice is founded depends on the opinions (editorials, lead articles, reviews, etc.) of high-profile leading clinicians.

● What do you think is the key problem with eminence-based health care?

■ Research findings are always open to interpretation. The interpretation by individual experts is subject to the bias of their interests and value judgements. Leading clinicians are likely to have strong opinions on their own interpretation of the literature or they may adhere to a historical precedent (how things have always been done).

The following example illustrates some of the problems associated with eminence-based health care. Cindy Mulrow (1987), a professor of medicine in Texas, USA, studied 50 narrative reviews by eminent physicians published in major medical journals between 1985 and 1986. She found that, although each review professed to offer an up-to-date and accurate interpretation of the research literature, the conclusions in 94 per cent (47/50) of these published reviews could not be substantiated on the basis of studies cited in each review article. One explanation for this outcome is that many eminent reviewers start with a conclusion and try (but fail) to substantiate this by referring to what they perceive as relevant and supporting literature.

Cause and effect

There is a danger that experts will use evidence as the means by which they can substantiate what they expect to find, and not look for other contributory factors. For example, following myocardial infarction (MI, the medical term for a heart attack), patients commonly develop irregular heartbeats (arrhythmias), often with fatal consequences because the heart muscle is damaged and the electrical conduction of signals within the heart is disrupted. You might therefore conclude that prophylactic treatment with drugs that reduce these arrhythmias (anti-arrhythmic drugs) should also reduce mortality, and that patients should be given such drugs on admission to a coronary care unit to avoid this complication. But evidence-based approaches that are focused on single cause-and-effect relationships run the risk of ignoring the multiple determinants of ill-health, as you will see in Chapter 8. Treating the symptoms of MI alone is unlikely to remove the underlying cause, which is often extensive muscular damage and continuing diminished blood supply to the heart.

Comprehensive research is more likely to produce research outcomes that quantify the relative risk associated with each determinant investigated, rather than making claims for a single 'cure'. That is, the outcome of the research will be an estimate of the relative risk associated with each determinant, taking into account all of the other determinants, and these figures can be used to investigate how each determinant might contribute to an overall reduced risk. Evidence on single aspects of disease often fails to provide the full picture, but attempting to take account of all of the multiple interacting determinants of ill-health can make rational decision-making more complicated.

From the previous discussion and your reading of Chapter 1, you can see that the use of research evidence in health-care decision-making is dependent upon certain conditions, and it is a consideration of some of these conditions to which we turn next.

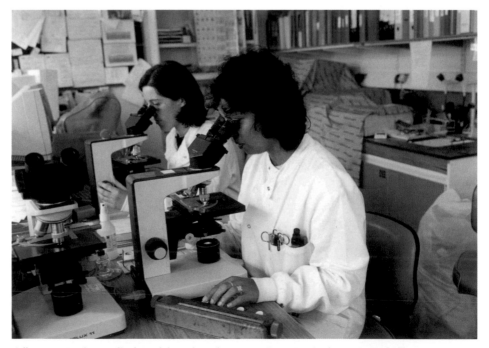

Adherence to the medical model tends to focus enquiry onto single cause-and-effect relationships. Microbiologists in a hospital laboratory search for the 'likely suspects' as causes of a disease process. (Photo: Mike Levers)

6.2   Research evidence as part of clinical decision-making

6.2.1 The research process

The quality of research evidence and how that evidence is prioritised in clinical decision-making is affected by the research process, including how it is funded.

Good evidence of the most effective clinical intervention for a patient with a particular condition is obviously important, and the first step in obtaining that evidence is identifying and clarifying exactly what is to be evaluated. In the model of rational decision-making outlined earlier, this is referred to as the stage at which the problem is identified (Figure 6.1, step 1). Assuming that there is agreement on what is the problem, then the next step involves establishing the criteria by which the evidence can be assessed. What this means is that the 'right' clinical questions need to be asked in order to produce the most useful evidence. Once these have been agreed, the research should be designed to take account of the following key elements:

1   the population/patient group of interest;

2   the type of intervention and potential alternatives;

3   the desired clinical outcome(s).

For example, estimates have been made that the health-care costs of obesity in a number of different countries ranged from 2 per cent to 8 per cent of the total health-care expenditure. For adults aged 16 or over in England in 1997, 17 per cent of men and 19.7 per cent of women were *obese* (a technical definition based on a body mass index, BMI > 30) (McIntyre, 1998).[2]

● Why is obesity considered to be an important condition in need of clinical intervention?

■ Obesity is associated with increased mortality and morbidity from cardiovascular disease, strokes and diabetes, as well as with mobility and respiratory problems.

The following example illustrates some key elements of research design.

In a typical English health authority of 500 000 people, around 397 000 are aged 16 or over, and of these around 34 000 men and 39 000 women are obese. Conventional treatment regimes include lifestyle interventions such as weight-reducing diet and exercise, which are notoriously unsuccessful ways of maintaining long-term weight loss.

Orlistat is a new drug, colloquially known as a 'fat blocker'. It was initially developed as a cholesterol-lowering drug, but weight loss in early animal studies suggested that the drug had anti-obesity properties. Researchers concluded that Orlistat may be a feasible strategy for the treatment of obesity.

The desired clinical outcomes are less straightforward, however. Orlistat was marketed as an adjunct to a diet regime to promote weight loss compared with a

[2] The BMI is calculated as the body weight in kilograms divided by the square of the person's height in metres. Energy intake, exercise and obesity are discussed in *World Health and Disease* (Open University Press, 3rd edn 2001), Chapter 11.

placebo[3] (a 'dummy' pill) in a two-year period. But the major impact of obesity needs to be considered on longer-term morbidity and mortality outcomes. Therefore, shorter-term weight loss is only a 'proxy' for longer-term outcomes, and begs the question of how valid and reliable the proxy indicator is.

The important question for clinicians and for health-service purchasers to ask is therefore 'to what extent will the weight loss provided by Orlistat lead to significant reductions in morbidity and mortality?' The reduction in morbidity and mortality is the clinical outcome, but the timescale and cost of supporting such long-term research may be prohibitive.

● Using all of these elements of the Orlistat example, formulate the research question that an evaluation study would have to answer.

■ The research question could be expressed as, 'Is Orlistat, combined with a weight-reducing diet for the treatment of obesity in people with a BMI > 30, more effective than a weight-reducing diet alone in reducing obesity-related mortality and morbidity?'

6.2.2 Funding research projects

Even when an effective clinical research question is formulated, the issue of funding needs to be considered. Who could or should pay for the study has an impact upon the quality of the research that is produced, and whether or not it proceeds. The production of good quality data that will produce rigorous evidence on the effectiveness of any clinical intervention involves experience, credibility, time, resources, good organisation and lots of effort from the researchers who plan the research study. Even then there is no guarantee that any individual piece of research will be funded. Indeed, in the UK the success rates of applications to various medical and health research funding agencies ranges between 1 in 2 and 1 in 25 (RDSU Grants, 1998). In other words, it is difficult to get research funded. So how do research commissioners select research studies to fund?

● What is most likely to drive the decision-making agenda on the evidence that needs to be collected and consequently what is most likely to receive funding?

■ Studies on the most cost-effective and efficacious strategies could provide the desired outcomes and save the most money while yielding the greatest benefit to patients, e.g. in the form of QALYs (Chapter 2). Studies that point to the need for greater expenditure may not prove so attractive to funding agencies.

Setting priorities

The Department of Health document *Research and Development for a First Class Service* (2000) lays out a development programme that meets the criteria of NICE and the priorities set out in the National Service Frameworks. In other words, the research and development that the NHS supports must be consistent with the 'NHS bodies' statutory duty of quality and their responsibilities for clinical governance' (Department of Health, 2000, p.5). However, the process of health research and development is not straightforward, as Figure 6.2 reveals.

[3] Use of placebos in clinical trials and issues to do with 'blinding' — the techniques for ensuring that patients, doctors and researchers do not know which patients took the active drug and which took the placebo, until the trial is over — are discussed in *Studying Health and Disease* (Open University Press, colour-enhanced 2nd edn 2001), Chapter 8.

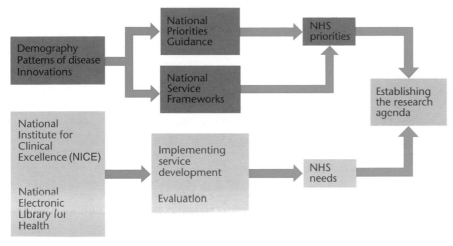

Figure 6.2   *Health research and development, policy and practice. (Source: Department of Health, 2000,* Research and Development for a First Class Service, *p. 25)*

Although it can be agreed that NHS priorities are determined largely on the basis of clinical and epidemiological need (e.g. cancers and cardiovascular disease have a high priority in the UK), as discussed in Chapter 1 they are also driven by political priorities, such as the emphasis in the late 1990s on primary care, the reduction of hospital waiting lists and historical precedents, such as high-status transplant surgery.

There is also a tension between the needs of the individual and the needs of the population as a whole. For example, the latest drug for the treatment of hair loss, a high-prevalence but low-severity condition, may be an important priority for some people without hair, but is likely to be less of a priority for health-care planners and public-health doctors. For them, the biggest threats to population health are cancers and cardiovascular disease, both of which are high-severity, high-prevalence conditions. Agreeing upon what constitutes 'the problem' is subject to competing interests that are often difficult to resolve despite apparently clear guidelines.

Once important clinical questions are identified, expressed clearly, and earmarked for research funding, consideration is needed on what sort of research should be commissioned, or alternatively the type and quality of evidence that should be produced (Step 2 in Figure 6.1). One form of research that is considered to produce good evidence is the subject of the next section.

6.3   Choosing the best: gold standards of research

A key determinant of the value of funded research will be its potential to influence clinical practice. To do that, the research must be considered rigorous, and able to stand up to critical appraisal by a clinician who is considering its value and relevance for her or his own clinical practice.

●   Read the fictional example of a randomised controlled intervention trial in Box 6.1 (*overleaf*) and suggest what might affect the *validity* of the results (i.e. does it actually measure what it set out to measure?)

Box 6.1   A randomised controlled trial of drug treatment X

A newly published research article proposes that drug 'X' for patients with asthma significantly reduced the number of acute attacks that led to their hospitalisation. The study was a randomised controlled trial (RCT). However, on examination of the process, you note that there were 1000 patients in the trial, of whom 500 were allocated to drug 'X' and 500 to a placebo. But of the 500 allocated to drug 'X', only 85 patients completed the study and were included in the data analysis, compared with 460 patients who completed the study in the placebo group.

■   It is important to ask what happened to the patients who dropped out of the experimental group. This high number of drop-outs in the drug 'X' group presents a problem. It could be due to the way in which the patients who were recruited to the trial were selected before they were randomised to one of the groups (a form of selection bias). Were there some unknown side-effects of drug 'X' that led to the huge number of drop-outs? In this situation, any data analysis that ignores the patients who dropped out is flawed, and consequently its findings are compromised.

6.3.1   Sources of bias

Bias inevitably creeps into most (if not all) evaluations. One way of managing bias in research studies is to be aware of all its potential sources and, if possible, to reduce it by good research design and adherence to principles of good conduct in research studies. Box 6.2 lists examples of different types of research bias.

Box 6.2   Sources of bias in research designs

- Two groups under comparison who are not from the same population (**selection bias**).
- Error on the measuring instrument (**measurement bias**).
- Unrepresentative sample (**sampling bias**).
- Clinicians, interviewers, assessors or patients selectively influencing results (study not conducted 'blind').
- Patients behaving differently *because* they are in a study.
- Patients not followed up for long enough to assess the outcome.

Selection bias is one of the most common problems in research studies, and can lead to flawed evaluation and poor quality evidence. For example, suppose that a study examined the benefits of vitamin supplements for pregnant women in preventing birth defects, and that two groups of women were studied: those that were *already* taking vitamins and those that were not. Then suppose that this study found that the women who were not taking vitamin supplements were more likely to have children with birth defects than the women taking vitamin supplements. The authors of the research study might conclude that vitamin supplements reduced the risk of birth defects.

● Explain why this is not a valid conclusion.

■ The two groups under comparison were not from the same population. One group of women consisted of those who had already decided to take vitamins, whereas the other group was not taking vitamins.

The two study groups can be referred to as **natural groupings** in that the subjects in each group shared a characteristic independently of the study. It is possible that other variables in the two groups could account for the difference in the birth-defect rate, such as smoking, diet, age and the number of previous pregnancies. Intervening variables such as these are known as **confounding factors** in research studies.

● Suggest how recruitment to an intervention trial could be planned in a way that would ensure that all of the control and experiment groups were as closely matched as possible.

■ One of the ways to eliminate selection bias is to *randomise* individuals from the same 'natural' population grouping to different study groups (i.e. allocate them at random to each group). In this way, it is possible to achieve in each group the same distribution of variables such as age, social class, previous obstetric history and any other confounding factors, including ones that the researchers may not have thought of.

Furthermore, to avoid bias by the people who measure the outcomes, the outcome criteria need to be clearly defined. Also, the people who make the measurements *ideally* should not be aware of who is receiving the intervention; similarly, the patients themselves should be unaware of whether they are receiving the experimental treatment, the standard treatment, or a placebo. This type of trial is said to be a **double-blind trial**.

Since it is not always possible to remove bias from studies altogether, researchers should acknowledge all sources of potential bias when they write their report of the outcomes. Furthermore, clinicians need to be aware of potential bias when they are appraising the quality of a published research study. After all, clinicians are able to use research evidence to benefit patient care only if they can distinguish good from poor evidence, or if a body such as NICE reviews all of the evidence for them and makes recommendations about best practice.

6.3.2 Hierarchy of levels of evidence

It follows that 'gold standards' for evaluating research are those research designs that minimise bias and maximise validity, *reliability* (i.e. the extent to which the same results are found if the same study is repeated), and relevance. To assist in the selection of good evidence (Figure 6.2, Step 3), the Centre for Evidence-based Medicine at the University of Oxford has ranked different types of study on the effectiveness of therapy and disease prevention, with the highest standards of evidence at the top, and those with the lowest reliability and validity at the bottom (Table 6.1 *overleaf*). This provides a **hierarchy of levels of evidence**. Similar hierarchies are also available for prognosis research, diagnostic studies, and economic evaluations (Oxford Centre for Evidence-based Medicine, 2001).

Table 6.1 A hierarchy of studies providing evidence of effectiveness in therapy and prevention.

Level of evidence	Ranking
1a	systematic review (with homogeneity) of RCTs
1b	individual RCT (with narrow confidence interval)
1c	all or none
2a	systematic review (with homogeneity) of cohort studies
2b	individual cohort study (including low quality RCT; e.g. <80% follow-up)
2c	'outcomes' research
3a	systematic review (with homogeneity) of case-control studies
3b	individual case-control study
4	case-series (and poor quality cohort and case-control studies)
5	expert opinion without explicit critical appraisal, or based on physiology, bench research or 'first principles'

Source: Oxford Centre for Evidence-Based Medicine (2001) University of Oxford, *Levels of Evidence and Grades of Recommendation,* http://www.jr2.ox.ac.uk/cebm/docs/levels accessed August 2001.

In Table 6.1, the term *homogeneity* (see 1a, 2a, and 3a) means a systematic review that is free of worrisome variations (heterogeneity) in the directions and degrees of results between individual studies. At level 1c, all-or-none criteria would be met for example if all patients died before the treatment became available, but some now survive with it; or when some patients died before the treatment became available, but none now die while being treated.

At level 4, a 'poor quality' study is one that failed to define clearly the comparison groups and/or failed to measure exposures and outcomes in the same (preferably blinded) objective way in both the comparison groups, and/or failed to identify or appropriately control for known confounding factors, and/or failed to carry out a sufficiently long and complete follow-up of patients.

Next, we will look at systematic reviews, which occupy the highest level in this hierarchy.

6.3.3 Accessing the evidence: systematic reviews

A **systematic review** is a rigorous collection, synthesis and interpretation of primary research evidence from a number of different studies, often from different countries. Such a review can only be as good as the quality of the individual studies it reviews. In examining the effectiveness of clinical interventions, the gold standard research design is the RCT, so a review of several RCTs represents the highest quality of evidence.

An important source of systematic reviews is the Cochrane Collaboration (already described in Chapter 2). This is a world-wide venture by clinicians and researchers to undertake and publish systematic reviews on important clinical topics. The Cochrane Database of Systematic Reviews (CDSR) also contains high-quality systematic reviews undertaken by other organisations, for example the NHS Centre for Reviews and Dissemination (CRD) at the University of York.

● What type of bias might exist in systematic reviews of *published* research findings?

■ Studies that find statistically significant benefits or harms are more likely to be published than those that find no significant effects.

This is called **publication bias**. In addition, **retrieval bias**, where poor literature searching leads to an increased possibility of important studies not being found, also presents problems, even though systematic reviews take systematic steps to minimise such bias. The next section considers how appropriate choices can be made of which evidence to collect.

6.3.4 Choosing standards: the suitability of the RCT

Evidence hierarchies such as Table 6.1 are a useful guide to the scientific value of different research designs. However, this does not mean that the designs at the top of the hierarchy should be used in all situations. For clinicians and service planners, the important question to ask is 'what level of evidence would be both *necessary* and *sufficient* to promote treatment and service changes that are appropriate responses to agreed 'problems'?' (Figure 6.1, Step 4).

The issue of what evidence is necessary for treatment and service change is especially pertinent in research into service delivery and organisation, where the population of interest to whom the intervention is directed is often a clinical department or a group of professionals, rather than patients. For most medical and drug research it is patients who are randomised to receive different treatments in an RCT. But if the intervention (for example, a service configuration change or an educational intervention) is in a department or professional group, then it is departments or professionals that must be allocated to alternative interventions.

● Why might it be practically difficult and/or inappropriate to apply the RCT methodology to departments and/or groups of professionals?

■ Rigorous research often requires large sample sizes, and it is difficult and often impractical to allocate entire clinical departments or groups of professionals randomly to alternative interventions. For example, randomly allocating 1 000 patients who all attend the same clinic, in the same year, to different drug treatments, is relatively straightforward, compared with the practical difficulties and cost of randomly allocating 1 000 hospitals from across the country to alternative service-delivery configurations.

Another problem with the use of RCTs would be the difficulty of preventing **contamination** between sites. For example, patients might visit different hospitals and the outcomes of care given to them in these settings could not be clearly separated. There will be too many influences on patient care that are specific to the culture and organisation of different hospitals to be able to allow for and measure their influence.

In such instances, it is important to consider not only what is practical, but also what evidence would be acceptable to policymakers and clinical decision-makers. For example, if it would cost £2 million to undertake an RCT involving randomisation of 50 hospitals, but the cost was considerably less for a comparative study between 10 hospitals involving in-depth qualitative data collection, then for the same amount of money many more research studies could be undertaken using the latter approach. In reality, it is more likely that RCTs will be used for clinical trials of drug therapy and less commonly for difficult practical interventions like surgery and/or process changes to service delivery.

6.3.5 Resolving competing interests

Making decisions about what is necessary and sufficient evidence is subject to competing interests, not only between decision-makers, but sometimes for individuals occupying dual roles. For example, how do the twin needs of evidence-based policymaking and cost management fit together? Both are the concerns of purchasers and providers of health care. But some health professionals occupy the dual role of purchaser and provider of health care (as discussed in Chapter 3). Furthermore, those on research funding bodies, and the reviewers who offer their judgements on the quality and value of a proposed study, are usually eminent researchers and scientists — not the patients and clinicians involved in delivering and receiving the intervention.

The way in which these decisions are made will reflect the process of resolving any competing interests. This resolution is likely to result in the most powerful interests being represented above those of less powerful groups and individuals (Chapter 1). Another 'competition' in health-care evaluation has often occurred between advocates of quantitative research, which is generally best suited to collecting evidence on the effectiveness of clinical products, and qualitative researchers whose methods have often been undervalued. One consequence of this is that research into health care as a *process* has been relatively neglected.

Evaluating the process of health-care interventions

Evaluation of the process of an intervention can extend our understanding beyond simple causal explanations. Studies may use a combination of quantitative and qualitative methods to generate data on the understandings of participants in what is taking place, the meanings that they give to practices and attempts to capture the subjectivity of an intervention. Process evaluations take account of the experience of health-care users and workers, and the wider political, economic and ethical structures that shape outcomes.

It is unusual for studies to focus on the process of care delivery, including the experience of patients. For example, the length of stay for some patients following surgery, or the recovery following a stroke, is more likely to be measured and also to inform policy and practice, than is the experience from the point of view of patients and their carers. (In Chapter 4, you heard about the lack of acknowledgement of informal carers.) The experience of patients following early discharge from hospital would require a different research approach.

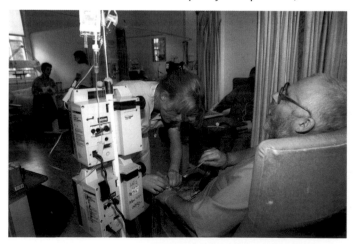

Post-operative care as a process of intervention is subject to formal and informal evaluation. The evidence from informal evaluation is often not documented or shared. (Photo: Duncan Phillips, Report Digital)

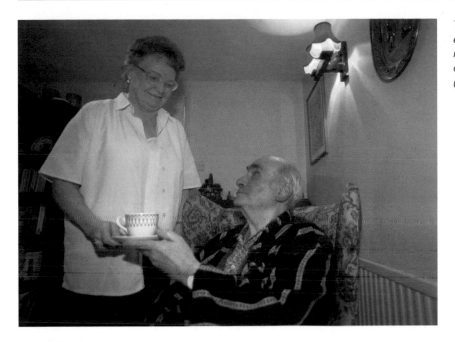

The evidence on the benefits of early discharge focuses on measurable outcomes more than on the experience of care. (Photo: John Callan/Shout)

● What type of data would be most suited to such an evaluation?

■ Qualitative data would be more likely to yield findings that contained information about the needs and priorities of the participants of the study, including the points of view of formal and informal carers.

The combination of both qualitative and quantitative data could overcome the lack of value that is attributed to research that is not considered to be gold standard. Quantitative studies usually involve larger sample sizes than are common in qualitative research, and the danger persists that more weight will be given to data on clinical outcomes from the larger quantitative sample. Whatever the nature of the study and method, its value will be based on both its own cost and its ability to evaluate the cost-effectiveness of the intervention. The cost of health-care interventions is the subject of the next section.

6.4 Costing the evidence

6.4.1 Ethical dilemmas in determining 'best value'

As well as considering the potential benefits and harms of a health-care intervention, it is important to know how much an intervention will cost. Evaluation will often include an element of economic assessment as an important component.

● Apart from the financial costs, what other costs need to be taken into consideration?

■ Costs also refer to *opportunity* cost, which takes account of any alternative use to which the resource might have been put (Chapter 2). Any comparison of cost-effectiveness would need to take into account an equitable distribution of resources.

The notion of affordability is important when resources are finite, but the dilemma is how to make the decision between treatment options (Chapter 2). A device for determining benefits is needed that takes into account opportunity cost. Several economic models for this have been developed.

● Suggest an economic model that allows a choice to made between two competing or alternative health-care interventions.

■ One model that was discussed in Chapter 2 is the quality adjusted life-year (QALY), which would provide a cost-per-QALY gained.

For example, consider the choice between hip replacement for patients who might live for a further 10 years and have a good quality of life, and a new drug for people with multiple sclerosis (MS) who might live for a further five years with a moderate or poor quality of life. The ethical case is stronger for supporting hip replacements over the new drug for multiple sclerosis if only one of these interventions can be afforded, and 'length of quality of life' is held to be the most highly valued outcome. But people who need hip replacements tend to be older than people with MS, which might tilt the balance in the opposite direction in some value systems and cultures.

The important point about comparisons between cost and cost-per-QALY gained is that this information is useful only if the decision-making framework and value system recognise this type of measure. If it does, then the research process would need to include data collection of patients' quality-of-life experience in the context of the prevailing culture.

6.4.2 NICE and the role of rapid reviews

In England and Wales, the NHS has moved towards a clear policy framework using cost-effectiveness evidence for particular health-care interventions. The National Institute for Clinical Excellence (NICE) was set up to provide guidance on particular health-care interventions (or technologies).

● Describe the role of NICE (look back at Section 2.7.5 if you are unsure).

■ NICE is part of the National Health Service (NHS), and its role is to provide patients, health professionals and the public with authoritative, robust and reliable guidance on current 'best practice'. The guidance covers both products and procedures (including medicines, medical devices, diagnostic techniques and procedures) and the clinical management of specific conditions.

Much of the work of NICE involves appraising the evidence for new pharmaceutical products, in which evidence produced by drug companies is examined. NICE also commissions appraisals through the NHS Research and Development Health Technology Assessment Programme. The Cochrane Collaboration's systematic reviews are held up as the highest level in the hierarchy of research evidence (Table 6.1), but they are expensive and time-consuming, often taking a year or more and the efforts of several people to complete.

Rapid reviews of evidence are urgent assessments considered as high priorities to the NHS and are prepared within three to six months of being commissioned, usually by the Health Technology Assessment Programme. Rapid reviews are a 'quick and clean' approach to health technology assessment, providing rigorous, protocol-driven appraisals of the benefits, harms and costs of particular interventions. Certainly in England and Wales at least, it seems that rapid reviews meet the criteria of being both necessary and sufficient for the work of NICE. It could be argued that rapid reviews are more valuable in the policymaking and decision-making arena, because they produce evidence *when* it is needed. Also, one characteristic of rapid reviews that does not appear in Cochrane Collaboration systematic reviews is the economic modelling of calculations of cost-per-QALY gained.

The timeliness and opportunity-cost savings afforded by rapid reviews compared with longer and more expensive systematic reviews needs to be considered. But here is the dilemma: is it worth paying the extra and waiting much longer to get a more robust answer, or is it worth taking the risk on accuracy in order to get an answer in time for a policy decision?

Another problem is whether treatments can be accurately costed in terms of benefits to patients, and whether this use of resources offers 'best value' to the population as a whole — as the following case study illustrates.

6.4.3 Beta interferon and relapse-remitting multiple sclerosis

Multiple sclerosis (MS) is a disease of the central nervous system. Its aetiology is not fully understood, although it is believed that MS is primarily an inflammatory condition where an autoimmune response ('anti-self') leads to destruction of the myelin sheaths that normally facilitate nerve conduction. (Myelin is a fatty substance wrapped like insulating tape around major nerves.)

The aim of treatment with *beta interferon*, a naturally occurring substance that modulates the activity of the immune system, is to slow down disease progression and to reduce the frequency and severity of relapses in patients with relapse-remitting MS (a form of the disease in which symptoms 'wax and wane' repeatedly). There are several different forms of beta interferon: the most researched is beta interferon 1alpha.

Although treatment and care of patients with MS is obviously an important health need, the condition has a relatively low prevalence compared with cancers and heart disease, so it may be given lower priority for research and evidence production. However, the potential cost of a new class of drugs for patients with MS — the synthetic beta interferons — ensures that there is substantial interest in their evaluation from policymakers, pharmaceutical companies, people with MS and their advocates.

Beta interferon has undergone clinical trials, and the evidence for its effectiveness is summarised by Nicholson and Milne (1999) who reported that, for every 100 people treated with beta interferon 1alpha, there would be, on average, 38 relapses prevented (range from 15 to 42). The *average* quality of life gained by these 100 patients would be 0.43 quality adjusted life-years (QALYs), with a range from 0.03 to 0.72, which indicates that some patients experienced virtually no benefit from the treatment, whereas others had some health gains. The calculation of the QALYs in this study was based on the assumption that during a relapse, MS patients decline from having no physical disability or problems with mobility or self-care to a situation where they have difficulty getting around the house, can go out only with assistance, and have major physical limitations.

It is also important to consider the cost-effectiveness of beta interferon.

- Beta interferon costs just under £10 000 per person per year, so for every 100 people treated, the cost is approximately £950 000 per year.

- The cost per relapse prevented (calculated by Nicholson and Milne) was £22 890.

- The cost per QALY gained by treatment was calculated at just over £2 million (with a range between £95 000 and £34 million estimated in a sensitivity analysis).

A decision on the affordability of beta interferon also depends on the opportunity cost of treatment. If, instead of spending money on beta interferon, these resources were used elsewhere to better effect, for example for specialist nurses, relapse care and mobility aids, then beta interferon is arguably less 'value for money' for people with MS.

● On the basis of the analysis by Nicholson and Milne, how would you sum up the evaluation of beta interferon as a treatment for MS?

■ Beta interferon appears to be a high-cost drug with limited clinical effectiveness for treating a low-prevalence condition.

In this chapter so far, we have discussed the dilemmas that arise from the evaluation of health-care decision-making. The debate has focused on the value of evidence used for evidence-based health care, but putting evidence into practice is not straightforward and we now turn to a consideration of some of the reasons.

6.5   Translating evidence into practice

Clinical guidelines provide guidance to clinicians and service planners on the treatment and care options for particular patient groups. For example, low back pain is a common condition, and clinical guidelines to GPs for its management include what to look for in the initial physical examination, together with the signs and symptoms that might indicate a serious condition, and what advice to give to patients about how to reduce the effects of their condition. But even if strong evidence is provided in support of clinical guidelines, it does not automatically follow that these will be implemented.

● What might be some of the constraints that prevent their take-up?

■ Doctors need to recognise that the guidelines are relevant and helpful to their practice. The example of the management of low back pain suggest that GPs would need to spend a lot more time on each consultation and this might not be possible within existing time constraints.

A systematic review of the uptake of clinical guidelines revealed that, if the guideline was produced 'internally', i.e. within the doctors' clinical base, then it was very likely to be adopted (Grimshaw and Russell, 1993). This poses a challenge for senior clinicians and managers faced with implementing locally the guidance emerging 'externally' from NICE.

6.5.1 Individual choice and collective responsibility

Although guidelines and appraisals might indicate to health-care staff those treatments and processes that will maximise good outcomes for patients, it is not surprising that patients may not agree with the presented evidence that a particular course of action is in their best interests.

An observational study, based on interviews with 260 randomly selected patients across eight general practices in the West of England, considered the impact of patient preferences on the treatment of atrial fibrillation — an abnormal heart-beat rhythm that is one (of many) risk factors for stroke (Protheroe *et al.*, 2000) Randomised controlled trials have demonstrated that patients with atrial fibrillation who are treated with an anti-coagulant drug (such as warfarin) have significantly reduced risk of having a stroke: this drug is specified as the treatment of choice in clinical guidelines (developed by Laupacis *et al.*, 1995; Lip, 1999). Despite the evidence of efficacy, there has been a low uptake of this treatment by patients. Perhaps patients managed in primary-care settings may be less willing to accept the side-effects of anti-coagulation, which includes the risk of bleeding, than the patients enrolled in clinical trials.

● What type of evaluation do you think would be appropriate in order to assess how patients make these choices?

■ A qualitative study analysing how patients decide would be likely to provide data on their reasons for refusing this drug.

Over 40 per cent of eligible patients in the atrial fibrillation study decided not to accept anti-coagulation treatment because of the side-effect profile associated with warfarin. This example illustrates one of the difficulties in translating evidence into practice. Regardless of the quality of evidence, treatment uptake is dependent upon patients being convinced that it is 'right' for them. Arguably, involving patients at the point at which treatment decisions have to be made is too late, but not all medical experts agree about the value of patient involvement earlier in the decision-making process.

Open University students should now read the article by David Sackett and colleagues entitled 'Evidence-based medicine: what it is and what it isn't' and Alan Maynard's reply to this in *Health and Disease: A Reader* (Open University Press, 3rd edn 2001). As you do so, answer the following questions:

● How do Sackett *et al.* present evidence-based medicine and what main criticism does Maynard make of their interpretation of what it means?

■ Sackett *et al.* state that evidence-based medicine is the integration of '… individual evidence from systematic research' and claim that this combination must include patient choice to militate against top-down guidelines being imposed. Alan Maynard's main criticism of the definition is that it is too focused on the individual patient and fails to take account of the cost-effectiveness of treatments. Maynard predicts that medicine that does not take into account equity and efficiency is one in which the middle classes will gain at the expense of 'poor' people.

A major dilemma for health-care evaluation, over and above dilemmas for individual patients faced with treatment choices, is how to achieve what traditionally has been referred to as **patient compliance** with an intervention, without crossing the line into coercion, while genuinely achieving informed consent. For example, what constitutes risk in childbirth has always been subject to debates about who has the right to choose and control the process (*see photo overleaf*). Recognition of this dilemma is reflected in the gradual adoption of a new terminology of **concordance** between the patient and the professional in achieving the 'best practice' intervention based on available evidence.

Risks for babies that are associated with water births are the subject of particularly heated debates about evidence showing that women's labours progress more quickly and they require less pain relief (Geissbuhler, V. and Eberhard, J., 2000) (Photo: Anthea Sieveking/ Collections Picture Agency)

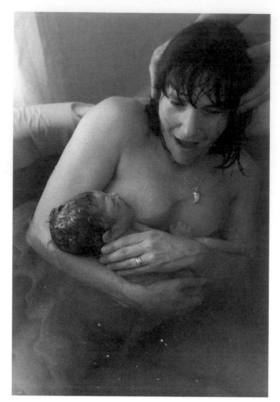

● Suggest examples of wider initiatives or interventions that override individual patient choice. How might scientists, public-health officials and politicians each be involved in such an intervention?

■ Examples could include mass medication decisions, such as fluoridation of water supplies, or spraying insecticides over geographical areas (for example, the chemical spraying of New York to prevent spread of the West Nile virus). Scientists provide the evidence, public-health officials apply the evidence, and politicians sanction the actions.

In these situations, some individuals are forced to comply who would not have chosen the intervention.

6.6   Conclusion: making the most of evidence

The evaluation of clinical practice as a rigorous process for determining clinical priorities also has to satisfy the potential end-users of the evidence. One form of evidence that will be increasingly required by health-care decision-makers is on the cost-effectiveness of treatments or care processes for particular patient groups. Such evidence helps decision-makers to 'grasp the nettle' and make difficult choices in allocating resources to different aspects of health care.

It is important to realise also that evidence exists in a social and human context. Not only does the uptake of evidence by clinicians and other health-care professionals rely on important local factors (as indicated by Grimshaw and Russell's work, 1993), but patients may decide not to follow the treatment or advice given to them for many other reasons. The question remains of how evidence-based practice can take into account the wishes of patients who do not base their choices solely on the efficacy of treatments, when measurements dominate clinical evaluation.

Likewise, the production of *local* evidence and the increased likelihood of the implementation of its findings cannot easily be generalised to wider populations, settings and practitioners. National guidelines might aim to produce quality, equity and efficacy, but if they are not relevant for local real-life situations, those responsible for putting them into practice won't follow national prescriptions.

The dilemmas highlighted in this chapter — difficult decisions concerning research priorities, evidence quality, affordability, implementation and patient choice — permeate the process of knowledge generation (research) and knowledge implementation (evidence-based health care). For any health-care system to make the most of its investment in research, these issues need to be acknowledged and debated.

OBJECTIVES FOR CHAPTER 6

When you have studied this chapter, you should be able to:

6.1 Define and use, or recognise definitions and applications of, each of the terms printed in **bold** in the text.

6.2 Discuss the main dilemmas posed by rational decision-making in the evaluation of health care.

6.3 Recognise and describe forms of bias in research studies and illustrate difficulties in demonstrating cause-and-effect links.

6.4 Explain why the systematic randomised controlled trial (RCT) is held to be the 'gold standard' in terms of health intervention evaluations and comment on its limitations and drawbacks.

6.5 Discuss the reasons for potential conflicts between evidence-based practice, local implementation of research outcomes and decision-making by patients about the uptake of treatment.

QUESTIONS FOR CHAPTER 6

1 (*Objective 6.2*)

The process of rational decision-making (Figure 6.1) is underpinned by assumptions. How do these impact upon the evaluation of evidence for clinical interventions?

2 (*Objective 6.3*)

In a comparative evaluation of two treatment options for depression, patients suffering from similar levels of depression as assessed by standard tests were randomly allocated to intervention groups A and B. Group A patients were given a new type of anti-depressant medication for six weeks, while those in group B attended six weekly sessions of individual psychotherapy. At the end of six weeks, patients in the two groups were assessed for their levels of depression, using the same tests. The assessment findings revealed that the patients in group A were much less depressed than the patients in group B. What further information about the studies would you need in order to assess the potential forms of bias that might have confounded the outcome?

3 (*Objectives 6.4 and 6.5*)

Why would it be impossible to use RCTs to evaluate how patients make treatment decisions?

4 (*Objective 6.5*)

Suggest some of the influences that impact upon the take-up of research findings.

CHAPTER 7

Medical technology: solving problems or creating dilemmas?

Study notes for OU students

This chapter builds upon your reading of *Medical Knowledge: Doubt and Certainty* (Open University Press, 2nd edn 1994; colour-enhanced 2nd edn 2001) which introduced you to the status of medical knowledge and the value that is placed on biomedicine. Chapter 9 of *Human Biology and Health: An Evolutionary Approach* (Open University Press; 3rd edition 2001) and Chapter 6 of the current book are both also relevant to this chapter. During Section 7.4.4 you will be asked to read an article by Andy Alaszewski and Ian Harvey, entitled 'Health technology and knowledge; the creation and management of uncertainty and risk' which can be found in *Health and Disease: A Reader* (**Open University Press, 3rd edn 2001**). There is also a television programme called 'Hospitals, who needs them?' which shows examples of the technologies used in the case studies in this chapter and presents views from the users' perspective.

The chapter is written by Carol Komaromy, the book editor.

You may also wish to read two optional reader articles 'Medicine matters after all', by J. P. Bunker and 'Doctor in the house: the Internet as a source of lay health knowledge and the challenge to expertise', by Michael Hardey.

7.1   Medical technology

The focus of this chapter is on the evolution of medical technologies and the dilemmas produced by their use. Opposing views of technological innovations present them as either the solution to all medical problems or the cause of continuous and escalating spending in the NHS. The reality is more complex and technology cannot be viewed in isolation from its wider social context (Chapter 1). As in any situation of change, the collective enterprise of introducing and using technological innovations in health care inevitably results in some degree of resistance and conflict.

The chapter begins by defining the term 'technological innovation' and presenting some of the key dilemmas that result from medical technologies. It then goes on to discuss the ways in which medical technologies are developed and controlled, and considers how technologies impact upon the structure and delivery of health care. Three case studies, magnetic resonance imaging (MRI), renal dialysis, and tele/cybermedicine, contextualise and illustrate the detail of dilemmas that result from specific medical technologies.

7.2   What are medical technological innovations?

'Innovations in medical technology' refers to several aspects of technology. **Medical technology** can be defined as the 'application of scientific knowledge to practical tasks'. In medicine, this includes both the *products* and the *processes* of health care delivery, as discussed in Chapter 6.

Process innovation in health care refers to new ways of organising and delivering care and includes for example, information management for transplantation and screening programmes, home care systems and day surgery.

Product innovation in health care refers to new ways of treating and detecting disease and includes drugs such as mood stabilisers, surgical procedures such as joint and organ replacement, and devices for detecting and diagnosing illness such as MRI and genetic testing. These innovations have vastly extended the *range* of conditions that can be treated effectively, the *type* of people who can be treated (including the unborn fetus), and hence the *numbers* of people who are potentially able to benefit from product innovations.

Once medical technologies are put into practice, they impact upon the system of health care as a whole and products and processes quickly become integrated. For example, the production and use of glucometers for measuring blood sugar levels has meant that people with diabetes can now control their own insulin medication more accurately and independently. This has impacted upon where and how their care is planned and managed. So the process innovation of the care of people with diabetes has changed as a result of this product innovation. Conversely, the process innovation of palliative care has as its primary focus the philosophy of placing the needs of dying people at the centre of decision-making. This has resulted in the production of new drugs and other products for the treatment of pain and symptoms.

The extent to which technological innovations shape the structures of health care is debated in Section 7.5, but the relationship between products and processes cannot be viewed in isolation from economic and political forces both inside and outside the NHS. Therefore an understanding of the dilemmas associated with technological innovations can only be gained by recognising some of the complexity of the structures that facilitate their development, and the changes that take place as a result of their adoption and implementation. In vitro fertilisation provides an example of this complexity.

7.2.1 In vitro fertilisation

A product and process innovation and one that raises a complex range of wider issues is that of in vitro fertilisation (IVF). Over 50 000 babies have been born as a result of IVF since the first baby was born in 1978[1].This involves an entire system of specialised care including drug treatments, the monitoring of ovulation using a sophisticated ultrasound scanner, obstetric, technical and counselling support and the provision of assisted conception treatment centres. Consequently, as at July 2001, IVF costs between £800 and £3 000 per treatment cycle. Each stage of IVF treatment includes an associated new product or process development and consequently, some of the dilemmas that result from IVF arise at several levels. The risk of multiple birth, which follows overstimulation of the ovary and the production of multiple eggs (ova), has to be weighed against the risk of failed fertilisation if only a single ovum is produced.

Table 7.1 presents data on the success rate of IVF treatment according to different causes of infertility.

Table 7.1   Clinical pregnancy and live birth rates for female causes of infertility in the UK, 1998–99.

Causes of infertility	Number of patients	Clinical pregnancy rate (%)	Live birth rate (%)
tubal disease	10 923	19.5	15.9
endometriosis[a]	3 194	21.9	18.2
unexplained	16 508	23.0	19.4
other	8 183	22.8	18.5

[a] Endometriosis is the excessive growth of cells both inside and outside the uterus, which often involves the ovaries.

Source: Human Fertilisation and Embryology Authority, 2000, *Annual Report 2000*, Table 4.3; www.hfea.gov.uk, accessed on 26 July 2001.

● According to Table 7.1, what is the most common cause of infertility among women treated by IVF, and what is the average success rate of all IVF treatments regardless of cause as measured by the pregnancy rate, and the range (the variation between the least and the most successful)?

■ The most common cause of infertility is 'unexplained'. The average pregnancy rate of IVF is 21.8 per cent and the range is 19.5 to 23.0 per cent. Note that the *live* birth rate is only 18 per cent on average.

[1] Some discussion of the issues surrounding access to IVF occurs in *Birth to Old Age: Health in Transition* (Open University Press, 2nd edn 1995; colour-enhanced 2nd edn 2001), Chapter 7.

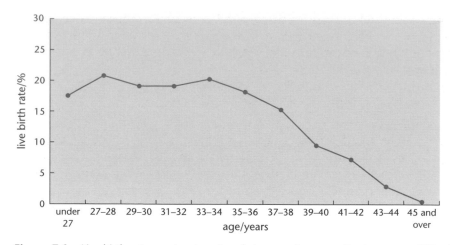

Figure 7.1 *Live birth rates per treatment cycle by age of women. Treatment was IVF using own eggs. (Source: Human Fertilisation and Embryology Authority,* Annual Report 2000, *Figure 4.2; www.hfea.gov.uk, accessed 26 July 2001)*

Figure 7.1 illustrates the success rate according to age. You will notice that from the age of 35 the success rate declines rapidly. Despite the many advances in reproductive technologies, the rate for women over 35 years is relatively low.

In the USA, all IVF treatment would be paid for at the point of delivery, but in the UK there is a debate about whether or not 'infertility' should be funded by the NHS. In order to qualify for treatment, 'problems' have to be acknowledged as medical ones, but what at first sight appears to be a dilemma that belongs in the medical domain has wider economic repercussions.

● What other cost needs to be taken into consideration in deciding what qualifies for NHS treatment?

■ The cost of providing one form of treatment means that resources are not available for something else. This is called the *opportunity* cost (Chapter 2).

If 'infertility' is defined as a medical condition, the question remains of whether resources should be allocated to the *treatment* of infertility, or to investigating the *causes* of infertility and thereby its prevention. (It is unlikely that there will be a simple causal relationship.) Even if IVF is offered by the NHS, difficult selection choices still have to be made of who qualifies for this expensive treatment and by what criteria they are selected. At the time of writing (2001), the government has requested that NICE (National Institute for Clinical Excellence) should evaluate IVF with a view to ending the 'postcode lottery' that existed throughout the 1990s.

● What further political, ethical and social issues does the example of IVF raise?

■ You might have suggested that there is an ethical dilemma about who has the right to reproduce and who does not, which underpins the high profile debate about the rights of older women, or women in same-sex relationships, to reproduce. There is also a political dilemma about who decides; this is illustrated by the government call for NICE to intervene in treatment decisions. The average number of embryos that were transferred was more than three, which increases the likelihood of multiple births, and has social consequences in terms of the additional support and services required for parents.

Concerns about child welfare are being raised increasingly within the debate about the ethics of reproductive technologies. The Human Fertilisation and Embryology Authority (HFEA) has been set up to regulate, license and collect data on fertility treatments and human embryo research in the UK. The potential for there to be 'fatherless' children born to mothers and an anonymous sperm donor threatens the security of the 'normal' family in popular culture.

The example of IVF illustrates that dilemmas about medical innovations are of different orders, and that medical technologies increasingly challenge traditional *biological* and *cultural* boundaries. Consequently, the use of some medical technologies produces emotional and ethical reactions that do not sit easily within the context of making rational 'scientific' choices.

The next section considers the extent to which it is possible for medical technology to provide benefits and raises some of the dilemmas that can result from their use.

7.3 Solving problems or creating dilemmas?

7.3.1 The success of medical technology

For many people, new drugs and surgical procedures have meant the continuation of a more or less normal life, particularly for those with chronic conditions such as diabetes and schizophrenia. For others, even if they cannot be cured, medical technology has meant a longer life. Table 7.2 provides examples of benefits to patients of treatments that have now become largely routine, but which were considered to be 'leading edge' innovations at their inception.

Most medical technologies are produced in response to medical problems with the hope that they will provide an effective solution, as Table 7.2 clearly demonstrates. When they are successful, new medical technologies have the potential to:

- expand the range of conditions that can be treated;
- increase the number of people who can be treated;
- identify the need for treatment more precisely;
- change the location and type of institution in which different treatments can be offered;
- change who can provide the necessary treatment.

Table 7.2 Some estimates of benefits to patients of medical technologies.

joint replacement	85–90 per cent pain relief; 70–80 per cent functional improvement
heart disease (revascularisation)	five-year relief of symptoms in 50–66 per cent of patients
peptic ulcer (drug treatment)	80–90 per cent healed in 4–8 weeks
unipolar[a] depression (mainly drugs)	70–80 per cent experience relief
cataract removal	75–95 per cent improvement in visual acuity

[a] Depression associated with extreme mood swings.

Source: Adapted from Bunker, J. P. (1995) Medicine matters after all, *Journal of the Royal College of Physicians*, **29**, No 2, March/April, Table 3, p. 109. (An edited version of this article appears in *Health and Disease: A Reader*, Open University Press, 3rd edn 2001.)

But necessity is not always the 'mother' of invention, and certain social, political and economic conditions need to be in place in order for innovations to be developed and adopted within a health-care delivery system. The IVF example illustrates that technology is not an activity that exists in value-free isolation, but rather is a social activity which has many constraints. As such, innovation is not driven by the scientific component any more than it is by the existing processes and structures within the health system that facilitate its use.

7.3.2 Creating dilemmas

The rise in degenerative disease in the Western world has resulted in an increasing need for certain sorts of treatment and a reliance upon medical technology to provide solutions. (The study of coronary heart disease in Chapter 8 illustrates this well.) This is partly driven by a medical focus on treatment rather than on prevention.

● Can you suggest other reasons why the historical *epidemiological transition* from a primarily infectious pattern of diseases to a predominantly degenerative pattern has driven the search for medical technological innovations?

■ Degenerative diseases are by their nature *chronic* (long-term), progressive disorders, that cannot be *cured* in the way that an infection *may* be cured by appropriate use of antibiotics. Nor do they get better 'on their own', as infections generally do in people with an intact immune system. So solutions must be capable of acting over many years to alleviate symptoms, slow down or reverse the inevitable deterioration. Moreover, entirely different solutions are required for different disorders (e.g. think about rheumatoid arthritis or Alzheimer's disease).

Providing solutions to chronic health problems impacts upon systems of health care and can make choices more difficult. The key dilemmas that result from the use of medical technologies include some of the following issues.

There are choices to be made between developing sophisticated high-cost medical technologies to treat a small number of people with varying degrees of success, and a more universal dispersal of health-care provision to a larger population. This competition for resources reflects a wider ideological and political division, making any compromise and resolution more difficult to achieve.

The speed of development in medical technology presents unique ethical dilemmas, which challenge existing professional and ethical codes and have the potential to erode patients' freedom of choice. The increase in 'living wills' in which people can request not to be officiously kept alive has arisen, in part, out of the prolongation of life beyond what some consider to be its useful term.

Attempts to control the risks associated with innovations can inhibit their production and act as disincentives to their further development. The need to maintain the growth of innovation has to be balanced against the need to stimulate growth — both of which carry risks.

Information as a form of power is shifting the boundaries of choice and control. This raises the question about how information should be controlled and by whom. Recent innovations in information and communication technology have challenged the role of medical experts and their ability to contain and control the quality and sharing of information (as a case study later in this chapter illustrates).

While it can be claimed that medical technologies improve the quality of life for many people, they are often only partial responses and not solutions. Renal (kidney) dialysis, which is considered in more detail in Section 7.6.2, provides a good illustration since it is a *treatment* for renal failure but not a *cure*. The reality is that only 30 per cent of the people who are treated by dialysis survive beyond five years (UK Renal Registry, 1999, p. 22).

Rather than saving costs, it could be argued that treatments for chronic conditions prolong people's lives and the subsequent need for supportive treatments including drug therapy. For example, Chandrasekar and colleagues (1999) record that the most commonly prescribed drugs in the USA are those for chronic conditions such as hypertension, depression, heart disease and arthritis. However, it remains the case that unforeseen consequences of medical technology can produce long-term damaging effects, and are one source of **iatrogenic disease**, that is illness caused by a treatment that is intended to cure, but which produces damage and hence the need for further health-care support. The development of medical technology provides part of the explanation for these dilemmas and this is the subject of the next section.

7.4 Growth management and sources of innovation

7.4.1 The development of medical technology

We have stated that the development of medical technology is influenced by more than the need to solve medical problems, and to understand its development it is useful to find answers to the following questions:

- Why did the development begin and why was it taken up?
- How was it funded?
- What is its application?
- What is its impact?

Ideas for research and development come from many sources, which include doctors who are pursuing 'own interest' research, drug companies and industrial spin-offs. Changes in health care or innovations are shaped and directed by funding choices, by policy decisions and by the need to control NHS spending as well as the need to provide solutions to health problems.

7.4.2 Sources of research and development funding

Much of the research carried out in UK hospitals is funded from public/private partnerships, with the private sector paying for equipment and supplies, while the public sector provides human resources — including the patients on whom new ideas can be tested. Much research is also carried out within private sector research laboratories, as well as academic institutions and facilities, some of which receive government funding through the Medical Research Council (MRC). In addition, private bodies such as the Wellcome Trust and the National Campaign for Cancer Relief are major investors in research in specific areas of clinical medicine. Table 7.3 (*overleaf*) presents the main sources of research and development (R&D) funding for health care and social care in England and Wales.

Table 7.3 Main sources of health-care and social-care R&D funding in England and Wales, 1998–99.

Government-funded research[a]	Department of Health	£360 million
	Medical Research Council	£296 million
	Health Education Funding Council Executive	£137 million
Non-government funded research	Charities[a]	£420 million
	Industry (mainly pharmaceutical)	£2 700 million

[a] Total research in health and social care funded by government and charities = *c.* £1 200 million.

Data compiled by Carol Komaromy from Department of Health Research and Development fact sheet, 'Research and Development in the Department of Health', November1999; www.doh.gov.uk/research, accessed 26 July 2001.

● From Table 7.3, who is the main provider of R&D funding? What percentage of health- and social-care funding is under direct government control?

■ The major provider of R&D funding is the pharmaceutical industry. The government provides, and therefore directly controls, three out of the five main R&D funding bodies in health- and social-care research and development. However, this accounts for less than a third of all funded R&D.

But, while it is clear that *all* R&D is dependent upon funding, the Department of Health regulations place clear controls upon private sector R&D, since it is in the NHS that most of the applications for medical technologies will be used. As you read in the previous chapter, evidence-based practice and evaluation criteria both tend to focus research grants more precisely on explicit outcomes and attempt to reduce the 'lottery' effects of research. This leads to another dilemma: should research funding be targeted in this way to produce best value from scarce resources, or does this stifle research creativity and the possibility of unforeseen breakthroughs in medical technology?

Since the early 1990s, NHS research has been subject to review and reform. Most notably the 1994 Culyer Report and in 2000 the NHS policy document *Research and Development for a First Class Service* (Department of Health, 2000h). The government regulates R&D through its 'First Class Service' policy. The extract from this policy in Box 7.1 illustrates how it fits into the wider agenda for health-care delivery.

Box 7.1 NHS Priorities and Needs R&D Funding

Responds to:

• National Priorities Guidance;

• National Service Frameworks (NSFs);

• National Performance Assessment Framework;

• National Institute for Clinical Excellence (NICE);

• Needs of the NHS.

(Department of Health, 2000h, p. 13)

Alongside these priorities, a new way of allocating funds for research was introduced in the 1990s to attempt to move the resources available for research away from large hospitals to community-based organisations, including general practice. The aim was to open up research opportunities to all health-care providers and to reduce inequality of access to research funds, while at the same time making research more directly relevant to the needs of the NHS. In these ways, the government has tried to modify the pattern of innovation, shifting the balance away from high to lower technology solutions. But, despite attempts to produce relevant and coherent research, the funding system has continued to operate in a competitive way, resulting in those with experience and sound reputations in research being more able to gain funding than newcomers. The pharmaceutical industry stands accused of being more interested in finding better drug *alternatives* to those of their competitors, rather than developing innovative new products (Rosenthal, 1993, p. 287). We now consider this industry in the context of the NHS.[2]

The pharmaceutical industry — a risky business?

In Table 7.3 you will have noted that industrial research into health and social care constitutes nearly one-third of R&D spending. In the UK in 1996, the NHS spent nearly 12 per cent of its total budget on drugs (Appleby, 1999). While it is recognised as economic 'wisdom' that if companies do not innovate they will lose their market share, it is also well known that the risks associated with innovation are high. Increasing regulatory controls have lengthened the time it takes for drugs to gain the approval they need in order to be marketed. The development cycle of a new drug, including its discovery, can last 12 years and only one-fifth of all drugs put forward for licences allowing their use on humans are approved. This is perhaps the major investment risk that the UK industry takes.

● What further product risks might damage the development of a new drug?

■ These might include:
  • being ineffective in treating the condition or illness under investigation;
  • producing toxic side-effects that are worse than the condition being treated;
  • not performing well in clinical trials;
  • not being a market success, e.g. because other drugs perform better or are more successfully promoted to doctors.

However, the development and the management of risk do not threaten the pharmaceutical industry in the UK as much as might be supposed.

● What makes the UK a special case in this respect?

■ The NHS provides regular and dependable customers, which gives the pharmaceutical industry advantages in this country that it does not enjoy elsewhere, in competitive insurance-based or fee-for-service health-care systems.

The authors of a study into the pharmaceutical industry claim that its success in the UK is related to the supply of well-qualified science graduates, government and charity-research funding, lower employment costs compared to other European countries and the concentration of the capital resources of major drug companies in the UK (Chandrasekar *et al.*, 1999, p. 74).

[2] The global aspects of the pharmaceutical industry, and in particular the product development priorities in relation to drugs for developing countries, are discussed in *Caring for Health: History and Diversity* (Open University Press, 3rd edn 2001), Chapters 8 and 9.

Whatever the success in business terms, however, patients are still exposed to risks associated with taking new drugs. In the 1950s, for example, the introduction of the drug Thalidomide for the treatment of morning sickness in pregnancy, led to babies being born with limb deformities. While all medicines used in the UK have to receive a licence before they can be introduced, their initial testing may be insufficient to reveal their full side-effects. The Medicines Control Agency was set up in 1989 in response to demands for more and tighter controls. But, there are risks associated with all new technologies and their management is the subject of the next section.

7.4.3 Policy controls and regulation

As Sir Alan Langlands, then Chief Executive of the NHS, stated in 1999, 'While the reasons for increasing demand are not fully understood, and are difficult to quantify, many believe that new technologies represent the single largest cost pressure' (Langlands, 1999, p. 1). An explicit aim of the government is to manage the supply and demand of health care.

Health Technology Assessment Programme

The NHS Health Technology Assessment (HTA) Programme was developed in 1993 in order to produce a coherent mechanism of control, with greater evidence of a needs-based approach. It is part of a tripartite research and development programme, the other two programmes being Service Delivery and Organisation, and New and Emerging Technologies.

Advisory panels on the HTA programme include representatives from the acute sector, diagnostics and imaging, methodology, pharmaceutical industry, population screening and primary and community care.

The declared aim of the HTA programme is:

> to ensure that high quality research information on the costs, effectiveness and broader impact of health technologies is produced in the most efficient way for those who use, manage and work in the NHS (Langlands, 1999, p. 1) .... Research carried out within the HTA Programme will support the work of NICE in developing national guidance and clinical guidelines. Similarly, access to the evidence base will be essential for the programme of National Service Frameworks. (Department of Health, 1999e, p. v)

In identifying service gaps, it is clear that the HTA programme will have a strong influence on what research assessment is commissioned. In supporting the work of NICE as part of clinical governance, which you read about in Chapters 2 and 3, the sanctioning of medical technology through formal assessment influences its development and implementation.

● Summarise the requirements of NICE and how this might serve to control medical technologies (if you are unsure, look back at Chapters 3 and 6).

■ NICE produces 'best practice' and evidence-based guidelines on medicines, medical equipment, clinical procedures and recommendations on where and for what conditions these should be used.

Since the process of appraisal takes about 12 months, NICE has the power to affect the period of time that it will take for treatments and procedures to be taken up. Appraisal is not the only form of control: once products are in use they need to be monitored and this is the role of a different government agency.

The control of medical devices

The Medical Devices Agency (MDA) is an executive agency of the NHS. It was set up in 1995 and its primary purpose is to:

> take all reasonable steps to protect the public health and safeguard the interest of patients and users by ensuring that medical devices and equipment meet appropriate standards of safety, quality and performance and that they comply with relevant Directives of the European Union. (MDA, 2000, p. 14)

The MDA aims to fulfil this role by:

> Negotiating, introducing and enforcing controls as set out in the European Medical Devices directives.
>
> Evaluating medical devices and publishing the findings.
>
> Investigating adverse incidents associated with medical devices. (MDA, 2000, p. 14)

● What is the potential difficulty with maintaining the quality of medical equipment?

■ You might have suggested that it is problematic for hospitals to purchase new products, even when the old ones are in need of replacement, so maintaining the quality of devices is often difficult.

It is only when equipment fails and an 'incident' occurs that the problem may become public. Furthermore, the increase in and variety among devices make competence in their operation more difficult to monitor and control. Finally, the system is dependent upon the co-operation of the staff who use medical devices. This suggests that the successful management of the tension between risk and innovation in medical technologies is easier during the development phase, but once in use their control is more complex.

7.4.4 Clinicians and the management of risk

The growth of technological products and processes in health care is driven by many separate forces. In the UK, the public institution of the NHS under direct government control is unique and means that the state controls aspects of research and development and monitors their use. But key groups, medical experts, government and the public have different interests and the unequal influence of these groups results in outcomes that tend to favour the most powerful.

Ulrich Beck, a professor of sociology in Munich, claims that doctors hold a special position since:

> Medicine alone possesses in the form of the clinic an organizational arrangement in which the development and application of research results to patients can be carried out and perfected autonomously and according to its own standards and categories in isolation from outside questions and monitoring. (Beck, 1992, p. 210)

Open University students should now read the article by Andy Alaszewski and Ian Harvey entitled 'Health technology and knowledge: the creation and management of uncertainty and risk', which is in *Health and Disease: A Reader* (Open University Press, 3rd edn 2001).

● What do Alaszewski and Harvey claim is the relationship between health technologies and uncertainty, and what is the impact of this upon the public?

■ They argue that, far from reducing uncertainty and risk, the increase in what it is possible to do through health technologies and knowledge corresponds to an increase in uncertainty. They claim that experts exploit this uncertainty to maintain and increase their control over the use of technology, and they offer the development of the specialism of radiology as an example. They also argue that perception of risk is influenced by 'fright factors' such as media representations, and that these are different from those which governments and experts claim as 'objective' risk assessments. This gap between official and lay assessment of risks presents itself as a sense of 'public helplessness' in the face of health technologies.

So far, this chapter has considered the way in which medical technology is funded and its regulation and control. But once technologies become part of health-care practice, they impact upon the way that care is delivered. We turn next to the introduction of *process* innovations.

7.5   Innovation and the structure of health care

7.5.1   Changes in treatment settings

Hospitals, particularly the major teaching hospitals, are engines for change in their own right, and devote part of their physical and human resources to the search for new forms of treatment, or to the underlying science which may eventually lead to many new forms of treatment. Within these hospitals, individual clinicians and teams often act as the champions of new procedures. Hospitals in the new millennium absorb more resources than ever, despite the shift towards primary care as the epicentre of the health service[3]. The decline in the number and size of hospitals since the 1990s is set to be arrested.

● The list in Box 7.2 is taken from *The NHS Plan*. Note what areas of investment have been given priority. How does it support the rhetoric of a shift to primary care?

■ The increase in hospitals and investments in hospital-care staff is set to increase alongside the expansion in primary care. Despite the rhetoric of primary care as the main health focus, it appears to be on course to continue to be secondary in resource allocation.

The continuing emphasis on hospital care and increasing specialism suggests that medical technologies will continue to develop in the twenty-first century. Changes in the demographic structure of the UK population, and the consequent increases in chronic conditions, have driven shifts to primary and community care. The management of many serious chronic conditions, such as asthma and diabetes, almost entirely outside the hospital has *further* secured the hospital as a site of increasing specialisms.

[3] The historical shift in power between independent practitioners, including modern GPs, and the hospital sector in UK health care, is described chronologically in *Caring for Health: History and Diversity* (Open University Press, 3rd edn 2001), Chapters 2–7.

> **Box 7.2   *The NHS Plan* 'pledges' for new investment**
>
> *Investment in NHS facilities*
>
> - 7 000 extra beds in hospitals and intermediate care;
> - over 100 new hospitals by 2010 and 500 new one-step primary care centres;
> - over 3 000 GP premises modernised and 250 new scanners;
> - clean wards – overseen by 'modern matrons' – and better hospital food;
> - modern IT systems in every hospital and GP surgery;
>
> *... and investment in staff:*
>
> - 7 500 more consultants and 2 000 more GPs;
> - 20 000 extra nurses and 6 500 extra therapists;
> - 1 000 more medical school places;
> - childcare support for NHS staff with 100 on-site nurseries.
>
> (Department of Health, 2000a, p. 11)

Since 1990 there has been a reduction in the number of hospitals of all sizes, certainly in comparison to the 1960s; the hospital of the new millennium treats many more patients but has fewer beds and much more of its clinical work is done on an outpatient or day-care basis. Both primary and tertiary care have expanded in response to a complex relationship between demographic change, medical technology and policy initiatives.

Tables 7.4 and 7.5 (*overleaf*) illustrate the shortening average length of hospital stay from 1981 to 1993 in England.

Table 7.4 Average length of stay (days) for ordinary admissions to non-psychiatric hospitals: England, 1981 and 1992–93.

	Average length of stay (days)	
Type of admission	**1981**	**1992/93**
non-surgical acute care	10.2	6.3
surgical acute care	7.5	4.8
geriatric care	66.1	23.5
maternity care	5.5	2.9

Source: Harrison and Prentice (1996) *Acute Futures*, King's Fund Publishing, Table 9.1, p. 129.

● Describe the trends in types of care in the data in Table 7.4.

■ For all types of admission, the average length of stay went down sharply between 1981 and 1992–93; the decline was greatest for geriatric care (down by two-thirds), and maternity care (down by almost a half), with surgical and non-surgical acute admissions staying for about two-thirds of the number of days in 1981. The trend in the reduction of the length of stay has continued, although the rate of decline was much less in the period between 1993 and 1996 (Appleby, 1999).

Table 7.5 Average length of stay (days) in non-psychiatric hospitals in England: selected conditions.

| | Average length of stay (days) | | | |
| | 1981 | | 1993 | |
	Males	Females	Males	Females
All	11.6	16.6	7.9	12.2
Infectious diseases	13.9	12.9	6.5	7.9
Malignant neoplasms	13.4	14.4	9.4	10.2
Benign neoplasms	7.3	8.1	5.1	6.1
Diseases of nervous system	37.1	54.4	20.3	33.9
Diseases of eye	8.6	9.4	3.3	4.0
Diseases of ear	4.1	4.5	2.2	2.4
Heart disease	13.7	30.6	7.0	12.0
Cerebrovascular disease	48.3	85.5	41.1	67.8
Diseases of respiratory system	14.6	28.4	10.9	18.9
Diseases of digestive system	7.9	10.2	4.8	6.3
Average length of stay for all settings, both sexes	22.32 days		9.37 days	

Source: Harrison and Prentice (1996) *Acute Futures,* King's Fund Publishing, Table 9.2, p. 130

● What striking feature do you notice in terms of gender in the data in Table 7.5?

■ The average length of stay for women is longer than that for men in all but one category (infectious diseases in 1981) — a division that did not change over this time period. The gender difference is more marked for some conditions (e.g. cerebrovascular disease) than for others (e.g. ear diseases), and the *size* of the gap has tended to get smaller over time.

We could speculate that since cerebrovascular disease tends to occur in older age groups and women have longer average life expectancy than men, they are less likely than men to have an informal carer at home. As you read in Chapter 4, home circumstances impact upon the ability to discharge people home 'early'. In Chapter 4 you also read that the shift of care away from the hospital to the community has also taken place for people with learning disability and mental health service users, and has resulted in the closure of many of the large institutions that once housed them.

● What new medical technology might have supported the closure of mental hospitals?

■ New psychiatric drugs enabled people with mental health needs to stay in the community with their illness relatively well controlled. In some ways, chemicals have replaced the physical confinement and control provided by long-stay institutions.

7.5.2 Economies of scale

The most advanced diagnostic equipment such as magnetic resonance imaging (MRI) scanners and facilities such as intensive care beds can only be provided economically in large hospitals with sufficient workload to guarantee that they will be fully used. These **economies of scale** make it progressively more difficult for smaller hospitals to maintain a full range of services or to offer the same standard of care as larger ones. As a result, the trend has been for smaller hospitals, and hospitals dealing with a specific group of patients such as pregnant women and children, to be closed in whole or part and their facilities transferred to larger ones. The expectation has been that as a result the quality of care will rise and the costs of delivering the services will fall.

The need for economies of scale drives the provision of tertiary care into an increasing concentration of specialised care. However, this is not the only driving factor: technology is a force in its own right and this is what we turn to next.

7.5.3 The technological imperative

One driving force that both sustains and increases technological developments is referred to under the umbrella term of the **technological imperative**, which holds that 'if it can be done, it should be done'.

Peter Freund and Meredith Maguire, both American medical sociologists, argue:

> The technological imperative implies that action in the form of the use of an available technology is always preferable to inaction. Indeed, once a technology becomes available, its use becomes almost inexorably routinised and considered standard. The failure to apply this standard care — no matter how inappropriate for the individual patient — would be reprehensible. The technological imperative is deeply embedded in many institutional responses to health crises. For example, most hospitals have created (and thus need to use) several high-technology wards, such as coronary and neonatal intensive care units, deliberately equipped and staffed to provide maximum multiple technological responses to patients' conditions. (Freund and Maguire, 1995, p. 243)

● The technological imperative raises serious ethical questions. Drawing on your knowledge of current events, suggest what some of these might be.

■ You might have suggested that demands for treatment can outstrip supply and result in difficult choices about who is entitled to receive treatment. You might have drawn on your knowledge from Chapter 6 to suggest an example similar to the following. The use of ultrasound scans at 12–14 and again at 20–21 weeks of pregnancy became routine in all hospitals during the 1980s and 1990s, without proper evaluation of the benefits of this technology. It then became *impossible* to evaluate, since there was no 'control' group of women who could be randomly allocated *not* to be scanned. Finally, the boundary between life and death is increasingly blurred by medical technologies that make it possible to sustain life without any obvious improvement in its quality, which raises questions concerning the value of extending the limits of medicine.

7.6 New technologies in health care: three case studies

This section presents three case studies which illustrate the function, development, application and impact of specific medical technologies and highlight some of the detail of the dilemmas presented in Section 7.3. As you read them, you should bear in mind both the dilemmas and also the impact of the technologies upon the way that health care is structured, the experience of patients and the extent to which their quality of life has been improved.

7.6.1 Magnetic resonance imaging[4]

The function of MRI

Non-invasive imaging, as a way of producing internal images of the body, began at the turn of the 19th century with X-rays, progressed into computerised tomography (CT scans, using a combination of computers and X-rays to produce more detailed and enhanced pictures), and developed most recently to non-ionising forms of imaging which do not cause damage to DNA. These non-invasive scanning methods include ultrasound and **magnetic resonance imaging** (MRI). Since the 1970s the use of MRI has become widely available and is now regarded as an indispensable diagnostic tool.

Parts of the body are exposed to a magnetic field inside a scanning machine and the image is produced by a computer which records information about the degree to which the atoms in different tissues 'resonate' (emit radio signals) in that magnetic field. Soft tissues such as the brain show up distinctly even when surrounded by bone (see Figure 7.2). Unlike X-rays, MRI scans do not involve potentially harmful ionising radiation.[5]

The chief advantage of MRI over X-ray and CT scanners is claimed to be its ability to produce detailed images of the characteristics of soft tissues; it is therefore considered to be the imaging technique of choice for soft tissue, neurological and muscular-skeletal disease. Another advantage is that in one single screening test it can provide more accurate information than would previously have been gained only by a combination of several other tests. Furthermore, unlike X-rays and CT scans, it does not expose patients to potentially harmful ionising radiation.

There are limitations to MRI, for example the lungs are full of air and do not give up a signal that can easily be detected. They are also sponge-like and contain a lot of small magnetic fields that destroy signals generated by the magnetic field and attempts are being made to overcome this. Recent techniques in visualising blood vessels by MRI require much less radio-opaque dye to be injected into the patient than is needed for X-ray pictures. In other words, the innovation of MRI is not a one-off development but something that is in a state of constant change and extension, even into areas to which it is not ideally suited.

[4] The TV programme 'Hospitals — who needs them?' has been prepared for Open University students studying this book as part of an undergraduate course. It illustrates the medical technologies that feature in these case studies. Students should read the associated *Audiovisual Media Guide* notes before watching the programme.

[5] Figure 9.3 of *Studying Health and Disease* (Open University Press, colour-enhanced second edition 2001) illustrates four different ways of scanning the human head.

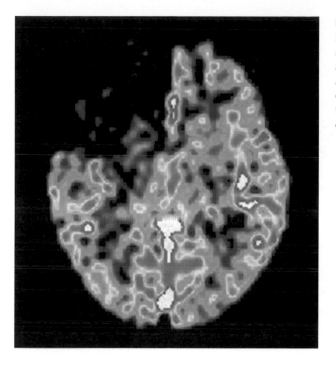

Figure 7.2 *An MRI image of the brain of someone following a stroke. MRI is most suited to producing images of brain and other soft tissue. This image shows how blood supply to part of the brain has been stopped by blockage of the artery. (Source: University of Nottingham, Division of Academic Radiology, www.nottingham.ac.uk/radiology/image_gallery, accessed on 26 July 2001)*

Development of MRI

MRI illustrates several features of technological growth. First, the scientific community did not decide to develop an instrument to solve problems associated with other forms of imaging. Instead the process, which began in the 1950s with nuclear magnetic resonance (NMR) spectroscopy, was incremental. Initially the magnets were so small that only small objects could be studied, and the first human examination was that of a finger.

Secondly, MRI was both an international and an interdisciplinary technology. It was developed in different settings, including the USA, UK, Finland, France, Japan and Germany, in different areas of disciplinary interest (physics, chemistry, biology and medicine) and in both a collaborative and a competitive way.

Thirdly, most of the funding for MRI research came from industry. In 1983 over 20 separate industrial groups were building NMR imaging systems. However, much of the pioneering work took place at Nottingham University in the UK, and by 1980 the Nottingham team had demonstrated the superiority of MRI over X-ray CT. The key patent for MRI was secured in Nottingham in the 1970s, but credit for its development is divided between the University of New York and the University of Nottingham.

The story of the development of MRI illustrates that the development did not follow a single linear path, but rather a collection of pathways with several innovations taking place in different disciplinary areas and geographical locations. While on one level the participants in its development were all hoping to achieve the same goal, MRI developed *both* competitively and collaboratively.

Applications of MRI

MRI is used in two main ways: as an emergency screening device and as an elective investigation that patients queue for (on a waiting list), usually as out-patients. Because of the large capital and running cost of MRI scanners, they have tended to be located in centres of expertise which have the resources to operate this system of screening.

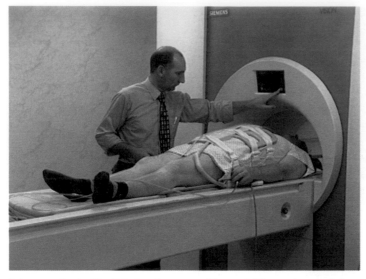

John, a patient with diabetes, is prepared for an MRI scan to search for a 'missing kidney'. For John, an MRI scan was a last resort prior to renal replacement therapy. (From TV programme 'Hospitals – who needs them?')

Hospitals are increasingly installing scanners at an average cost at the time of writing in July 2001 of £10 million each. Thus MRI use is driven by both clinical and economic utility. This produces another contradiction in its potential and actual use, because to make them cost-effective MRI scanners need to be used as much as possible, in other words their economic effectiveness (cost per scan) depends upon economies of scale. Also, because new generations of faster and more accurate MRI scanners are being developed, current machines have a limited life expectancy of 5–7 years. Furthermore, because MRI is mainly used as a last resort, people who are not classified as being in need of emergency screening might undergo a range of tests *before* they receive an MRI scan. This form of use contradicts its potential advantage as a single replacement for a series of tests.

A study undertaken at Queens Medical Centre in Nottingham assessed the value of MRI scans in the first hour of people who are suspected of having had a stroke, and illustrates the potential of MRI (Moody, 2001). For example, MRI can detect irreversibly damaged brain tissue much earlier than CT scanning and therefore allows for a more appropriate treatment regime. It is particularly important to be able to distinguish patients who have a clot in a main blood vessel supplying part of the brain from those who have had a haemorrhage; in the latter case, the use of 'clot busting' drugs would increase bleeding with potentially fatal consequences. It is also important to be able to predict those people whose brains have the potential to recover following treatment and thus avoid unnecessary treatments.

Dilemmas in the use of MRI

Part of the current system involves the need to make decisions about how the use of MRI is rationed. At the moment, only demands for emergency MRI are met and non-urgent cases are put on a waiting list, using the classical triage system (Chapter 2).

● Waiting for screening has potential costs. What are some of these costs?

■ If disease can be detected more accurately and treatment provided early, then waiting for screening tests is a false economy. Even people with non-urgent chronic conditions might need to receive treatment for symptom relief (e.g. for pain) while they are waiting for a diagnosis.

Secondly, the sophistication of MRI has a potential deskilling effect on technicians and clinicians who interpret imaging information, because part of their professional skills are replaced by the capabilities of the technology. But increasingly detailed pictures of body tissue increase the amount of information available about the human body and this makes it more difficult to distinguish between normality and abnormality. Professor Alan Moody, an expert in medical MRI, describes these dilemmas thus:

MRI is a dual-edged sword with regard to the resolution and diagnostic ability that it provides. The images are getting clearer and clearer, which ... [can] make diagnosis easier and easier. We can manipulate the sequence to make pathological processes look more obvious than the normal surrounding tissues, so it could be said that MRI will put radiologists and clinicians out of business because anyone would be able to make a diagnosis. In some situations that would be true, in some situations that will be false .... As well as providing better pictures the anatomy becomes more difficult to understand as more structures are made visible. Trying to differentiate what is normal structure from an abnormal structure, what is an artefact on the picture — something that's been made by the machine itself — all become extremely important to understand why they're here, and whether they're important. As the techniques advance the pictures will become clearer, the information will become clearer but there'll be more of it that will need interpretation .... (Moody, 2001, quoted from the associated TV programme, 'Hospitals — who needs them?')

Finally, the technological imperative clearly drives MRI development. The need to keep up to date with the latest technology and economies of scale has created the demand for increasing numbers of better and bigger machines. More accurate images lead to demands for this level of accuracy in more screening investigations. In this way, what it is possible to do with this technology creates its own escalating demand. However, this demand for more accurate information is not necessarily met by the ability of medical staff to treat newly diagnosed conditions.

7.6.2 Renal dialysis[6]

The function of renal replacement therapy

Renal dialysis, often called **renal replacement therapy** (RRP), is used for patients with 'end-stage renal failure' and replaces part of the function of their failed or failing kidneys. The kidneys perform a vital life-sustaining function by filtering waste products and fluids, controlling blood pressure and producing a hormone called erythropoitin. This hormone is responsible for the production of red blood cells in the bone marrow, without which people become anaemic[7]. Dialysis replaces part of the kidney function by eliminating waste products from the body.

There are two main types of dialysis, haemodialysis and continuous ambulatory peritoneal dialysis (CAPD). **Haemodialysis** involves attaching people via a blood-line to a dialysis machine through which their blood is filtered for about four hours, two or three times a week. Because regular venous and arterial access is needed, a surgical procedure to insert a shunt, called a fistula, into a large blood vessel is performed. This fistula sometimes fails so that new access is needed.

One-third of people who receive dialysis for renal failure will go to a hospital renal ward or a satellite hospital several times a week for haemodialysis. Another one-third of people will manage their own haemodialysis at home using a home dialysis machine and technical support when necessary. However, septicaemia is a relatively

[6] The associated TV programme shows dialysis machines in use in two different settings — a renal dialysis unit in a large hospital in the centre of London and a unit in someone's home.

[7] Mutations in the gene that codes for erythropoitin are discussed in another TV programme for Open University students, 'Blood lines: A family legacy?'

common side effect; a blood infection contracted through the fistula, which consequently requires hospital admission for a course of intravenous antibiotic treatment. Therefore, hospital in-patient care is a regular feature of renal dialysis.

Continuous ambulatory peritoneal dialysis (CAPD) relies on the peritoneum as a semi-permeable membrane to filter waste products from the blood and drain fluid into and out of the abdomen. Fluid is introduced to the abdominal cavity via a fistula created by minor surgery into the patient's abdomen (the peritoneal cavity) on the other side of the peritoneal membrane and draws off excess salt and water in a process of osmosis[8]. About three litres of fluid are infused and left in the abdomen for up to six hours and then drained off and discarded before being replaced by another load. This dialysis takes place either three or four times a day and each exchange takes 30–60 minutes. About one-third of dialysis patients manage CAPD independently at home. Some patients dialyse overnight using a simple pump. As with haemodialysis, the risk of infection is high and one of the possible side effects of this form of dialysis is peritonitis, a serious infection of the peritoneum that requires hospital admission and intravenous antibiotic treatment. If that happens or if CAPD fails for other reasons, patients have to undergo haemodialysis until CAPD can be resumed. If they return to this form of dialysis, another fistula has to be formed.

Both haemodialysis and CAPD are dependent upon the availability of emergency hospital support.

Development of renal dialysis

The initial development of dialysis machines was directly driven by clinical need. Early treatments for renal failure used a form of purging in which patients were given high doses of laxatives, resulting in waste products being filtered out across the membrane of the bowel. Early dialysis was only successful for reversible renal failure. There were two key problems which had to be overcome. The first was that because there was no effective anti-coagulant available until the 1940s, blood taken

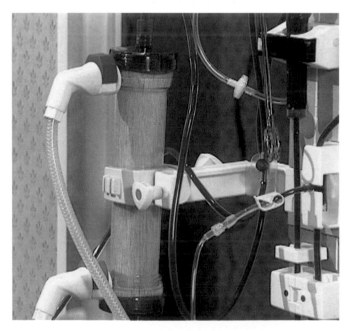

from patents clotted in the tubing and dialysis machine. The second was the difficulty of sustained access to blood vessels and it was not until the 1960s that the first successful shunts were used.

Dialysis was largely a Western development, and the first successful dialysis machine was used in 1943 (by a Dutchman, Professor Houston, living in Nazi-occupied Holland). The first dialysis units were set up in the UK in 1960s. Dialysis machines of this period were large and the membrane consisted of blocks of metal

The transparent plastic tube reveals the synthetic, semi-permeable membranes that filter the blood. These act as artificial kidneys. (Photo: TV programme 'Hospitals – who needs them?')

[8] The movement of fluids and small molecules across semi-permeable membranes under osmotic pressure is described in *Human Biology and Health: An Evolutionary Approach* (Open University Press, 3rd edn 2001), Chapter 3.

sheets which had to be chemically sterilised between use for 7–10 hours, making them cumbersome and difficult to use. Many improvements have been made to dialysis machines since they were first introduced. Most have been in blood access, anticoagulants (anti-clotting agents) and the quality of the filter membrane in the dialysis machines. Also, the quality of the fluid used in dialysis (of 120–180 litres per session) has improved dramatically.

Application of renal dialysis

The main causes of renal failure are autoimmune disease (in which the person's immune system attacks tissues in the body) and systemic disease, of which diabetes is the most common. The incidence of end-stage renal failure increases with advancing age and therefore older people account for an increasing percentage of those who are treated. For example, the average age of people in the UK on dialysis in 1980 was 45–50 years, and in 1999 it was 60–65. Haemodialysis is an expensive treatment and is the second most expensive intervention (in the NHS, only drugs used to delay or treat AIDS are more costly).

- What is one of the most obvious consequences of this increased demand for dialysis?

- With finite resources increased demand means that rationing decisions have to be made.

Dialysis requires specialist units and staff and involves the need for 24-hour cover by technicians for hospital and home treatment. There are costs to individual patients of time, inconvenience, discomfort and the need to keep to a strict dietary and drug regime, as well as the need for support from both formal and informal carers.

Information about renal dialysis has only been centrally collected in a renal register database since 1997, and of the 75 renal units in England, Scotland and Wales only 36 contribute to the register, so the data in Figures 7.3 and 7.4 (*overleaf*) are incomplete. They show the number and percentage of patients receiving different forms of treatment modality for end-stage renal failure, by age.

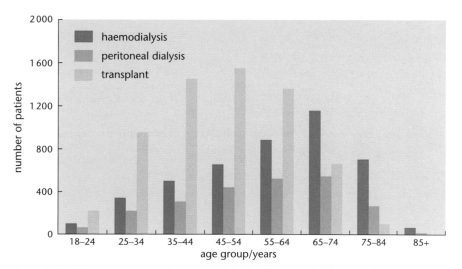

Figure 7.3 *The number of patients treated by the three modalities in each age group. (Source: UK Renal Registry, 1999, p. 32)*

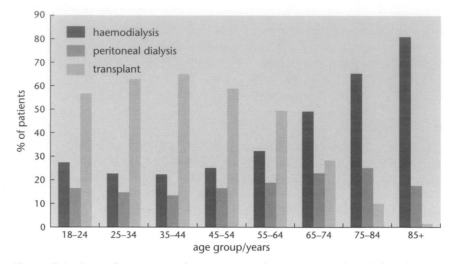

Figure 7.4 *For each age group, the percentage of patients on each modality of treatment. (Source: UK Renal Registry, 1999, p. 32)*

● In Figures 7.3 and 7.4, what are the most striking features of the relationship between age and treatment modality?

■ There is a predominance of transplantation in younger patients, whereas older people are more likely to receive haemodialysis than CAPD.

CAPD treatment is complex and older people are more likely to be judged as less able to manage this treatment independently.

Dilemmas in renal dialysis

In 1998, the Renal Registry recorded 1 229 deaths from end-stage renal failure or its complications, and 1 788 new patients. In 1997–98, the registry estimated the growth in increased demand for renal dialysis to be 5.6 per cent.

● What factors could affect decisions about the type of treatment people in end-stage renal failure are offered?

■ Your list might have included things like:
  • availability of different forms of treatment in a locality;
  • demand for those treatments locally (e.g. some parts of the country have higher proportions of older people);
  • costs of different forms of treatment, including support services;
  • patients' ability to learn to manage treatment;
  • the ability of the NHS to offer training to patients;
  • convenience to and preference of patients for one form of treatment over another;
  • impact on the patient's quality of life.

The appropriateness of continuing dialysis treatment for people who have many other chronic conditions associated with ageing is difficult to assess. In May 1996, the Department of Health published the results of a national survey of renal units in England, which confirmed that older people were less likely to receive renal replacement therapy than younger people.

Figure 7.5 illustrates the proportion of different age groups of people in renal failure who were accepted for renal replacement therapy.

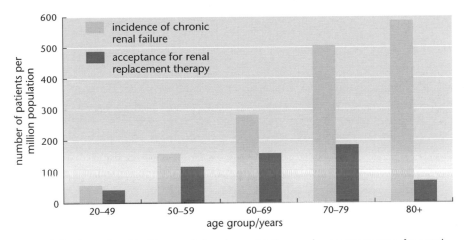

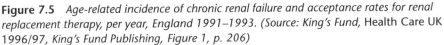

Figure 7.5 *Age-related incidence of chronic renal failure and acceptance rates for renal replacement therapy, per year, England 1991–1993. (Source: King's Fund,* Health Care UK 1996/97, *King's Fund Publishing, Figure 1, p. 206)*

Bill New and Nicholas Mays, two senior researchers then at the King's Fund, claim that:

> The clear implication is that as one gets older the likelihood of contracting chronic kidney failure increases but the chance of receiving treatment decreases. This is not the result of an explicit NHS policy, just the result of clinicians making difficult decisions in the context of limited budgets. Nevertheless, to Age Concern this constitutes a *prima facie* case of discrimination against elderly people. (New and Mays, 1998, p. 206)

The Department of Health estimates dialysis treatment costs for patients on haemodialysis to be £29 000 per year per patient and about half as much for CAPD. One of the main concerns for hospitals is the cost of specialist staff for the dialysis unit and also of transporting patients long distances to large general hospitals. One result of these constraints has been the development of treatment at smaller local hospitals (satellite hospitals) for haemodialysis and the encouragement of patients to perform their own peritoneal dialysis at home. But treatment at home shifts the costs to the community setting. The technological imperative operates to increase demand for dialysis.

For patients, the combination of treatment and travel to hospital can take up most of the day and can be quite exhausting. There is a waiting list for home haemodialysis and CAPD, and the patient's home must accommodate all of the machinery and supplies of dialysis fluid; ideally it should have a room put aside for treatment and storage. Whatever the setting, the demands for support are high and, regardless of the type of treatment, the number of people in need of dialysis outstrips supply and rationing decisions have to be made about who should receive treatment. This means that people will die in renal failure because they are not offered treatment.

Furthermore, the type of treatment that patients are offered can be complicated by what is available in terms of support so that the patient's preferred choice might not be an option. Because the NHS works on a 'first come first served' basis, it is more difficult for doctors to decide to omit treatment (Chapter 2). It is certainly very difficult to withdraw dialysis once it has been started.

The demand for emergency haemodialysis remains high; there has to be enough spare treatment capacity to provide it to people who go into renal failure unexpectedly and also to those patients for whom CAPD fails either temporarily or permanently. But the complexity of dialysis treatment makes the needs of patients difficult to predict. When one form of treatment fails, another has to be offered immediately since without treatment someone in renal failure would die in a matter of days.

Medical technologies have meant that 'expertise' can be programmed into machines to such a sophisticated level that patients can now manage complex forms of treatment and monitor their condition relatively independently. The shift of the location of medical knowledge is the subject of the third and final case study.

7.6.3   E-health: telemedicine and cybermedicine[9]

The function of E-health

Advances in information communication technology (ICT) are integral to the development of MRI and dialysis in that both are supported by computerised (software) instructions, monitoring and data analysis. Changing the way that knowledge is organised and accessed impacts upon how health care is delivered. Making information accessible to everyone with web or Internet access has the potential to change the power relationship that exists between patients and medical experts. 'E-health' as a form of electronic access to expert opinion has the potential to revolutionise care systems and challenges geographical boundaries of where health care and expertise is located. Procedures such as radiology, endoscopy and all forms of medical monitoring have the potential to be carried out in the primary care setting rather than having to be based in acute hospitals.

Development of telemedicine

Telemedicine can be defined as a system which uses telecommunication to transmit medical information and services. The exchange of health-related information in a digital form includes verbal advice, X-rays, pathology slides and medical records. The information can be transferred in 'real' time or can be 'stored and forwarded'.

The telecommunication systems and the Internet are not new developments nor were they developed in response to a health-care need. They are part of the infrastructure of societies world-wide, although the degree to which they are taken up in the population varies between countries and access is often dependent upon individual wealth. The adoption of these systems for the use of health care has been in the process of development for at least the past 40 years.

Simon Wallace is a medical consultant for a telemedicine organisation and claims that attempts to establish telemedicine in the 1960s and 1970s failed for three main reasons: the costs were too high, the images that were produced were of a poor quality and the service structure and trained staff were not in place (Wallace, 1998).

●   How would you explain the recent increase in the interest in telemedicine?

■   One of the reasons for the renewed interest in telemedicine is that it fits the criteria of access and equity. It is also has the potential to become financially beneficial because the 'expert' who will interpret the data that is being produced need not be physically present at the screening test or the consultation.

[9] The TV programme shows examples of telemedicine and cybermedicine and some projections of its future use.

Figure 7.6 illustrates one example of telemedicine in the UK. Secondary care is general hospital care while tertiary care is that which requires highly specialised hospital skills and technology.

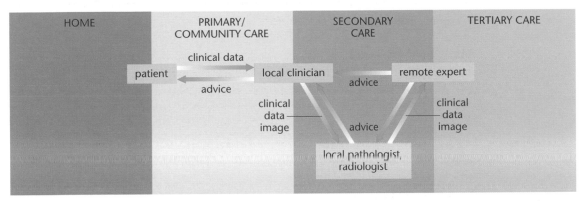

Figure 7.6 *Telemedicine — telepathology and teleradiology. This Figure shows how in remote settings, or those without access to the appropriate medical specialist, information can be sent via a telephone line to an expert at a distance. Local doctors, pathologists and radiologists can discuss results with the expert, in the presence of the patient. (Source: Wallace, S., 1998, Telemedicine in the NHS for the Millennium and Beyond, in Lenaghan, J. (ed.) 1998,* Rethinking IT and Health, *Institute for Public Policy Research, London, Figure 4.1, p. 59)*

Telemedicine is an unusual intervention in that it separates the care provider from the patient, but one important aspect is that the information remains within the control of medical experts.

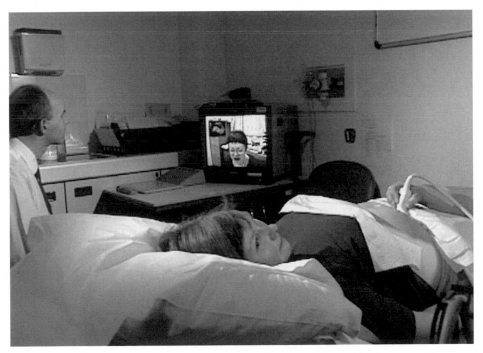

This pregnant woman has been spared the stress and inconvenience of having to travel a long distance for a detailed scan of her baby. The scan images are sent to an 'expert' in interpreting them, based at a large general hospital. (Source: TV programme, 'Hospitals — who needs them?')

Application of telemedicine

The telemedicine industry is world-wide and has been growing rapidly in the past decade. As in Figure 7.6, the introduction of telemedicine allows the resources of large general hospitals to be accessed 'from a distance'. Thus doctors in secondary hospitals can send images electronically to colleagues in tertiary units and consult them about a diagnosis. Similarly GPs or doctors working in the community can engage in joint consultation with experts in distant locations via television links. Some nurse-run minor injuries units are linked to hospitals in this way, allowing the nurses to access advice if they are not sure whether they can treat the patients presenting to them. At the moment, these developments have not gone far enough to transform the way that care is delivered and for the most part, telemedicine is applied to curative medicine. But the potential for major change exists.

The following list in Box 7.2 shows some of the medical applications of telemedicine.

Box 7.2   Examples of applications in telemedicine

Teleradiology — distant interpretation of radiological images.

Telepathology — distant interpretation of pathology specimens.

Teledermatology, teleophthalmology, teleoncology, telecardiology, telepsychiatry — distant consultation in different clinical specialisms.

Telecare and telemonitoring — advice and monitoring a patient's condition in the home.

Telesurgery — advice between an operating theatre and a remote expert during a surgical operation.

Telerobotics — computer-assisted surgery and clinical applications of virtual reality.

(Lenaghan, 1998, p. 60)

In comparison with MRI and RRT, telemedicine, because it is used in health care by medical experts (Chapter 6), is dependent upon evidence from evaluation. The examples of telemedicine in Box 7.3 illustrate this.

These two different examples give some idea of the range of possibility for applying telemedicine and also show that the products and processes, i.e. hardware system, the quality of information transmitted and the patient's experience all need to be evaluated. As discussed in Chapter 6, rather than there being one key evaluation question, there are several. Each aspect of the innovation impacts upon the nature of this new form of communication, so that the innovation is both complex and multifaceted.

● Why should information that people access from the Internet be considered different from that gained from other sources?

■ The Internet is global and the information exchanged is limitless. Unlike more conventional forms of publishing, there is no way of monitoring the quality of information since anyone can publish on the Internet.

For example, cybermedicine puts the idea of medical expertise being owned and controlled by medical experts under serious threat[10].

[10] If you have time, an optional article in *Health and Disease: A Reader* (Open University Press, 3rd edn 2001) addresses this point: 'Doctor in the house: The Internet as a source of lay health knowledge and the challenge to expertise' by Michael Hardey.

> ### Box 7.3 Examples of telemedicine
>
> *Minor Injuries Service: London — Belfast*
>
> A live telemedicine link was established between a nurse-led minor injuries clinic at the South Westminster Health Centre in Central London and the Accident and Emergency department of the Royal Victoria Hospital in Belfast. Nurses could obtain immediate real time advice from a medically qualified specialist. In the first 10 months of operation, approximately 1 in 200 cases (49 in total) were seen using the telemedicine link. Preliminary calculations suggested that the use of a low-cost telemedicine link was extremely cost-effective in comparison with conventional medical cover.
>
> (Lenaghan, 1998, p. 91)
>
> *Teledermatology in the Highlands of Scotland*
>
> A telemedicine video-link was established between the main hospital in Inverness and the medical centre on the Isle of Skye 120 miles away. Weekly clinics were held seeing 2–5 patients and lasting 60–90 minutes. A total of 51 patients were seen during 15 clinics over 5 months. A fax of the referral letter was available and a written opinion by the consultant provided after each consultation. The diagnosis was able to be made in most cases with over half the patients satisfactorily dealt with via this medium. However, many patients felt that despite the advantage of immediate consultant opinion, it would be more appropriately used as a review technique.
>
> (Lenaghan, 1998, p. 95)

Cybermedicine

Cybermedicine is a form of global medical knowledge and a system of dissemination and access and is likewise both product and process innovation. Cybermedicine includes health education, self help, information dissemination and support groups.

Gunther Eysenbach and colleagues further distinguish **cybermedicine** from telemedicine by claiming that in cybermedicine, 'there is a more global exchange of open, non-clinical information, mostly between patient and patient, sometimes between patient and physician and between physician and physician' (Eysenbach *et al.*, 2001, p. 459). Cybermedicine is usually part of preventive medicine and public health.

Other definitions of cybermedicine include the use of computers in general and 'futuristic' visions of the human body, or what has become known as cyborgs: bodies which are part-machine, part-human[11].

Dilemmas of E-health

It is difficult to establish the right balance between the use of remote medicine and health care that is delivered 'face to face'. The benefits of being able to 'consult' at a distance and exchange medical information focus on convenience and cost savings. This is certainly helpful to patients who are at a distance from medical expertise, but medical experts might find that being available for an increased number of consultations or 'on call' for advice, increases rather than decreases their workload.

[11] A cyborg of the human heart is shown in the TV programme 'Hospitals — who needs them?'.

In telemedicine, the relationship between doctors and patients is based upon the assumption that the only valuable information is that which can be transferred remotely. Some people would argue that there is more to medical encounters than the exchanges of 'scientific' information, for example, doctors may miss subtle clues or patients may feel unable to confide in a TV monitor — while others would claim that a 'remote' encounter is more liberating for the patient. The dilemma lies in being able to offer a choice of consultation to those who would benefit most from either. Providing the choice of how to consult and how to receive information is part of patient autonomy and this is arguably as important as the quality of information being exchanged.

Security concerns, because of the potential increase in remote access to medical records, require there to be encryption methods in place for data security. But, regardless of the success of encryption, anxiety that can result from the perceived lack of confidentiality can outweigh the benefits offered by this form of exchange.

Cybermedicine is much more difficult to define as a single technology and to locate geographically and therefore to regulate and control. Apart from issues about the quality of information, an increase in inequality of access to health can result in some people being advantaged over others. There is also the potential for the 'worried well' to demand more time from health-care professionals as a consequence of information they obtain from the Internet.

Some members of the health professions are critical of the diversity of this information, claiming that it is potentially confusing to lay people. There is, however, contrary evidence which suggests that users are quite capable of discriminating between conflicting information. For example, Michael Hardey, a medical sociologist who conducted a study into the use of health information, claims that not only are users able to discriminate between conflicting information, they appear to welcome information about non-orthodox approaches to health (Hardey, 1998).

7.7 Conclusion

The case studies have allowed you to consider the detail and complexity of the use, development, application and dilemmas in established and emergent medical technologies. What is clear is that their development trajectories have shared a relatively slow beginning prior to their adoption. It is as if medical technology acquires its own momentum, partly driven by the technological imperative, but also by a need to justify the investment in development and subsequent economies of scale. While each intervention has gone some way to solving problems, its use has created further dilemmas.

This chapter began with a claim that medical technological innovation is both a solution to medical problems and part of the problem. E-health raises the question of whether challenges to the power of medical experts will be eroded or will further increase current inequalities in health.

The sociologists Mike Featherstone and Mike Hepworth argue that:

> … the faith of modern societies in scientific and technological process, the idea of an upward curve of development inevitably transporting us in the direction of a better world, has a religious quality to it. It [technoscience] contains powerful images of how nature, the human body and the social world can be re-made and reconstructed. (Featherstone and Hepworth, 1998, p. 163)

Featherstone and Hepworth ask if it will be possible to overcome the limitations of the human body. Their answer is that technology is both a part of society and also transforms society. In other words, technology and social life are in a dynamic relationship. This chapter and Chapter 1 have shown that technology, per se, cannot solve medical problems, neither does it act alone to create continuous and escalating NHS spending. Rather, how it is used and controlled within health care provides important information for understanding its role.

OBJECTIVES FOR CHAPTER 7

When you have studied this chapter, you should be able to:

7.1 Define and use, or recognise definitions and applications of, each of the terms printed in **bold** in the text.

7.2 Discuss some of the major research and policy measures that government in the UK has used to control the growth of medical technologies in recent years.

7.3 Recognise and illustrate the impact of both product and process innovation upon the structure and delivery of health care.

7.4 Use specific examples of medical technology to demonstrate the extent to which each succeeds in solving specific medical problems but creates new challenges to the health-care system.

7.5 Discuss the key dilemmas that result from the introduction of medical technologies in health-care practice, using examples taken from this chapter.

QUESTIONS FOR CHAPTER 7

1 (*Objective 7.2*)

The ability to support cost-effective innovations in health care is not straightforward. What are some of the difficulties that governments face in controlling spending on new medical technologies?

2 (*Objective 7.3*)

What type of innovation is IVF? To what extent does the technological imperative explain the introduction and increasing use of IVF?

3 (*Objectives 7.3 and 7.4*)

'Innovations allow people to have more choice about health care.' Evaluate this statement.

4 (*Objective 7.5*)

'Medical technologies such as MRI were developed to reduce the risks of existing technological interventions.' Critically assess this statement.

CHAPTER 8

Preventing disease: the case of coronary heart disease

Study notes for OU students

This chapter refers back to the detailed discussion of the contribution of age, gender, ethnicity and social class to patterns of health and disease in the UK, which you studied in Chapter 9 of *World Health and Disease* (Open University Press, 3rd edn 2001); problems in establishing a causal association between Western diets and heart disease were discussed in Chapter 11 of that book.

During Section 8.4.3 of the present chapter, you will be asked to read an article by Ann Bowling in *Health and Disease: A Reader* (Open University Press, 3rd edn 2001), entitled 'Ageism in cardiology', which was optional reading for an earlier book in this series. We also refer to a debate in the Reader, 'Should smokers be offered coronary bypass surgery?' which is set reading for this chapter.

This chapter was jointly written by (in alphabetical order) Eric Brunner, Senior Lecturer in Epidemiology at University College London Medical School, Basiro Davey, Senior Lecturer in Health Sciences, Department of Biological Sciences, The Open University, Harry Hemingway, Senior Lecturer in Epidemiology at University College London Medical School and Director of Research and Development at Kensington and Chelsea and Westminster Health Authority, and Carol Komaromy, Lecturer in Health Studies, and Moyra Sidell, Senior Lecturer in Health and Social Welfare, in the School of Health and Social Welfare, The Open University.

8.1   Introduction

It is often said that 'prevention is better than cure' and it might seem self-evident that prevention should be the preferred strategy in combating disease. Common sense tells us that it must be better to try to prevent misfortune rather than have to deal with its consequences. But in the realm of health care this is a far from simple matter, as the case study of coronary heart disease (CHD) demonstrates later in this chapter.

First we consider the dilemmas that affect the issue of preventing ill health more generally.

The first and overarching dilemma lies in deciding the desirable balance between prevention, treatment and cure. Where resources are finite, expenditure on disease prevention within the formal health-care system is likely to divert funds from treatment services. Given the choice, should we shift the emphasis away from those who are already sick in order to preserve or increase the future health of those who remain well?

Trying to determine where the priorities should lie takes us into another contested area beset by uncertainties about the relative effectiveness of different prevention strategies. Developing *appropriate* and *acceptable* strategies to prevent disease and demonstrating their clinical and cost *effectiveness* is not a straightforward matter. As discussed in Chapter 6, demands for evidence-based medicine and the renewed focus on evaluation make it increasingly unlikely that disease-prevention initiatives without an effective evaluation strategy would be supported by public funding.

However, many of the strategies to prevent disease pose serious problems for evaluation. This may be because they entail very long-term social, behavioural or environmental changes, or because the 'outcomes' involved cannot easily be defined and measured, or because it is difficult to control for influences external to the strategies themselves. So there is a dilemma to be resolved here about what factors to measure and in what populations, and what weight to place on the outcomes.

A third dilemma arises from the tension between individual freedom and social control. To what extent are preventive strategies socially or morally justified? Strategies to prevent disease can restrict individual freedoms (as in the banning of smoking in public places or the compulsory wearing of seat belts), or exert coercive pressure that may arouse guilt over 'unhealthy' behaviour. Such strategies can reach into every aspect of people's daily lives – in their homes, workplaces and communities – and inevitably they focus yet more attention on health and disease. This may be beneficial in encouraging people to become more aware of their health, but it may also have negative effects, such as the anxiety caused when screening is imposed on fit and healthy people. This ethical dilemma is especially acute where disease-prevention strategies lack clear scientific evidence to justify their implementation.

A fourth dilemma hinges around the question of who is responsible for health. Is it the individual, the community or the agencies of the state? Without a clear understanding of and agreement on what determines ill health it is difficult to locate responsibility for its prevention within specific agencies.

A former Chief Medical Officer, Sir Kenneth Calman, distinguishes the determinants of health into the five categories in Box 8.1. If factors such as the environment, employment, transport and education partly determine people's health, then responsibility for health cannot just lie with the individual – it also has to be the

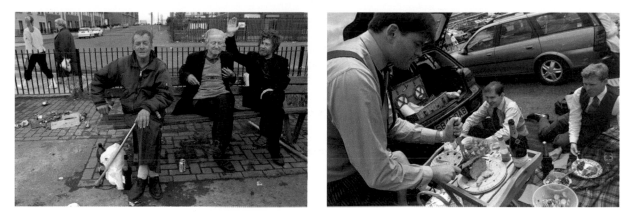

A park bench on an estate in Possil, Glasgow, and a scene in the car park at Ascot racecourse. Is it ethically justifiable to ban alcohol consumption or smoking in public places as a disease-prevention strategy? Or would reducing poverty have greater impact? (Photos: John Harris/ Report Digital; Jess Hurd, Report Digital)

responsibility of several agencies. Indeed, demands for action based on the evidence of inequalities in health have risen to the top of the world agenda, putting responsibility on governments to reduce the gap between the best and the worst health profiles within and between nations. (We discuss strategies for tackling health inequalities in the UK in Chapter 9 of this book.)

Box 8.1   Determinants of health

- Biological factors, such as ageing and genetic influences.
- Social and economic factors, such as education, housing, employment, income and poverty, and cultural aspects.
- The environment, including the quality of the air, water and soil, transport, climate changes; including infection.
- Lifestyle issues, such as diet, smoking cigarettes, drug abuse, alcohol and physical fitness.
- Health services, and the way they are delivered and accessed; including developments in medicine, diagnostic techniques, and rehabilitation (Calman, 1999, p. 284).

Later in this chapter we explore the dilemmas outlined above and their consequences from the perspective of coronary heart disease. But first we will examine what is involved in disease prevention at a more general level.

8.2   Strategies for preventing disease

In this chapter we have chosen to focus on **disease-prevention strategies**, which concentrate on preventing or at least reducing the effects of specific diseases. They represent part of a much wider **health promotion** agenda, which seeks to promote positive health through the development of healthy public policy, strengthening community action and creating supportive environments for health. This very broad agenda is in harmony with the 'new public health' initiatives of the 1990s onwards, and is discussed further elsewhere.[1] Here we demonstrate how great are the complexities involved in the superficially simpler area of disease prevention.

8.2.1 A hierarchy of disease prevention

Disease-prevention strategies can be loosely classified into three levels according to the type of activity they involve:

1 **Primary prevention**: strategies that aim to prevent the onset of disease. This category includes most types of immunisation. But strategies aimed at inducing changes in the behaviour of individuals are also a major component of primary prevention; for instance, changing diet to lose weight, taking up exercise and, of course, giving up smoking, are all ways in which individuals are encouraged to reduce the risk of a whole range of diseases, such as lung cancer, diabetes and CHD. Primary prevention is often informed by screening for risk factors that may predispose people to develop a disease later in life unless action is taken now – an area of great interest in the prevention of CHD, as you will see later. Determining the extent of risk associated with a certain predisposing factor, devising an effective means of changing behaviour and demonstrating that the outcomes are cost-effective is a hugely difficult task.

2 **Secondary prevention**: strategies that aim to detect and cure a disease at an early stage before it causes serious irreversible problems. Screening of tissues or body fluids provides important diagnostic evidence, for example in the early detection and treatment of certain cancers, particularly of the breast, cervix and prostate gland; the identification and control of diabetes; or the detection and treatment of certain infections, such as tuberculosis. However, screening to detect disease raises the dilemma of whether this is always in the patient's best interests; for example, mass screening by chest X-rays to detect lung cancer was carried out after World War II, but was abandoned when it became clear that detecting most such cases 'early' had no impact on the length of time that people survived.

3 **Tertiary prevention**: strategies that aim to minimise the effects or reduce the progression of an already established irreversible disease, for example, the multiple drug therapies that have delayed the progression to AIDS in people infected with human immunodeficiency virus (HIV). Here the overlap with treatment is hard to disentangle. Some would include hip replacements or heart bypass surgery in this category, but many would claim such procedures are curative interventions rather than preventing the progress of the disease. Another example is palliative care which aims to relieve symptoms such as pain or nausea for people with terminal illness, but again this classification is debatable and many would put such interventions in the treatment category.

● Give an additional example of a disease-prevention strategy at each of the levels outlined above.

■ There are many you could have chosen from, but here are some examples. Primary prevention strategies include sex education in schools aimed at reducing teenage pregnancies, abortion and sexually-transmitted infections. Secondary prevention includes paediatric assessments performed on newborn babies to

[1] The 'new public health' movement is discussed in an earlier book in this series, *Caring for Health: History and Diversity* (Open University Press, 3rd edn 2001), Chapter 7. For those who would like to pursue it further there is another Open University course devoted entirely to health promotion: K301, *Promoting Health: Skills, Perspectives and Practice*.

detect and treat biochemical abnormalities such as phenylketonuria (PKU)[2], or physical problems such as cleft palate or 'clicky' hip joints. False teeth could be categorised as tertiary prevention in that they minimise the irreversible effects of tooth loss from decay, and so could 'nerve blocks', the surgical procedures to alleviate chronic pain.

The focus of much disease prevention is on the primary and secondary levels, where the distinctions between prevention, treatment and cure are easier to distinguish. In addition to screening methods (discussed in Section 8.3), they depend substantially on the twin approaches of health education and health protection.

8.2.2 Health education

As in the example of sex education above, **health education** is an important disease prevention strategy in that it aims to give people the knowledge and skills to change potentially health-damaging behaviour. Health education operates at many levels. At the face-to-face level many health professionals engage in health education in their day-to-day encounters with their clients. GPs, practice nurses, community nurses and health visitors routinely provide advice and information about diet, exercise, alcohol, drug use and smoking. Health education is also to be found at a group level, for example in campaigning or special interest groups, and in locally focused leaflets and posters in doctors' and dentists' waiting rooms. At a national level we are all exposed to mass media campaigns that often use shock tactics to inform and warn individuals about the dangers of drinking and driving for instance, or unprotected sex. In whatever form they take however, health education messages are directed at the individual whose behaviour they seek to change.

● Taking into account the different determinants of health set out in Box 8.1, what is the main drawback of a strategy that focuses on individual action?

■ It ignores the social context in which individual choices are made and the social and environmental influences on health. This approach also runs the risk of 'blaming the victims' by holding them responsible for their own illness.

Keith Tones, Professor of Health Studies at Leeds University, however, has been a long-term advocate and defender of health education (Tones, 1993). He claims that it has the potential to empower individuals by giving them the knowledge and skills to take control of their own health. Nevertheless it is clear that many of the factors that affect people's health lie in the social and economic environment and there is a limit to the extent that individuals can take charge of their own health. This requires tackling inequalities (which is the subject of the next chapter), but health-protection measures are also important.

8.2.3 Health protection

Health protection involves legislation to protect public health. Examples include health and safety legislation in the workplace, the work of the Food Standards Agency in assuring standards of food hygiene and safety, the monitoring of air pollution from industrial sources, and protection from sewage washed up on beaches.

[2] PKU is a rare disorder of protein metabolism, for which all newborn babies in the UK are screened by testing a 'heel-prick' blood sample; the biology, cost-effectiveness and ethical issues raised by screening for this condition are discussed in *Human Biology and Health: An Evolutionary Approach* (Open University Press, 3rd edn 2001).

● Can you think of other health-protection measures that legislate at the level of individual behaviour?

■ Seat-belt legislation is one example; bans on smoking in public places are another.

Health protection that affects personal behaviour is resisted by certain groups of people who claim that it infringes individual liberty. The same grounds for opposition have been raised in the campaign against fluoridation of drinking water, because no-one is exempt from such 'health protection' and opponents accuse the state of public health 'paternalism'. Balancing individual freedom against the potential benefits to society is a dilemma that the introduction of health-protection measures has to negotiate.

It is notable also that the introduction and enforcement of health-protection legislation is generally accompanied by substantial health-education campaigns.

8.2.4 Summary

The boundaries between treatment and prevention are not always easy to distinguish; nor is it straightforward to categorise a particular strategy as operating at the primary, secondary or tertiary levels. The strategies involved in health education and in health-protection programmes may also interact. However, given these provisos, the categorisation discussed in this section provides a useful framework within which to consider specific approaches to disease prevention.

● Categorise the types of prevention given in Table 8.1 as either health education or health protection, and primary or secondary prevention. Then complete the empty rows 1, 3, 4, 5 and 7 in the third column to indicate where responsibility for taking action lies.

Table 8.1 Examples of activities aimed at preventing disease.

Aim of the prevention strategy	Intervention	Responsibility for implementation
Statutory		
1 Reduction in cigarette smoking	higher tobacco taxation	
2 Prevention of waterborne disease	provision of safe water supply	water companies
3 Reduction of road traffic accidents	breathalyser	
4 Prevention of food-borne disease	inspection of food premises	
Voluntary		
5 Reduction in cigarette smoking	education in schools	
6 Reduction in coronary heart disease	advice on reducing fat in diet	health professionals, health promoters
7 Prevention of measles	immunisation	
8 Reduction of invasive cervical cancer	screening	doctors, NHS Trusts, health authorities

Based on Royal College of Physicians (1991) *Preventive Medicine: A Report of a Working Party of the Royal College of Physicians*, RCP, London, Table 1.1, p. 6.

■ Interventions 1 to 4 are all examples of health-protection measures; 5 and 6 fall into the territory of health education; 1–7 operate at the level of primary prevention (i.e. preventing disease or disability from occurring), whereas 8 is secondary prevention, because it detects and then treats the early stages of a disease. To complete column 3 you might have suggested the following:

1 government

3 police

4 local authority inspectors

5 health promotion workers, teachers

7 doctors, nurses and health visitors.

8.3 Screening for disease

Screening has been described as:

> ... the practice of investigating apparently healthy individuals with the object of detecting unrecognised disease or people with an exceptionally high risk of developing disease, and intervening in ways that will prevent the occurrence of disease or improve the prognosis when it develops. (Farmer and Miller, 1983, p. 4)

Screening is a medically driven strategy for disease prevention. It relies on tests involving medical technology and expertise, and any action taken on the test results is usually a medical responsibility. Within the NHS, screening tests are still largely aimed at detecting signs of a particular disease or risk factor; it is unusual to find the type of 'general health screening' offered in the private sector, where a whole battery of tests is performed on the same individual to build up a detailed health profile.

Screening tests may be designed to detect physiological changes that commonly happen before the onset of a particular disease (contributing to *primary prevention* if the disease can thus be prevented), or to detect an early stage of the disease itself (*secondary prevention* if the disease can be treated more effectively than if detected later). For example, screening to detect and reduce a risk factor such as raised blood cholesterol may result in the primary prevention of CHD (the subject of Section 8.4), whereas screening to detect and treat microscopic breast cancers is secondary prevention. Cervical screening for so-called 'pre-cancerous cells' falls somewhere between the two, because it is not known what proportion of these cells would revert to normal or progress to cancer if left untreated.

The dilemma about screening is, as we said earlier, whether it is cost-effective at preventing disease; it cannot simply be assumed that more screening tests applied to more of the population will inevitably result in worthwhile health gains for individuals, or represent the best use of resources for the population as a whole.

8.3.1 Principles of effective screening

In 1968 Wilson and Jungner produced ten criteria for effective screening for the World Health Organisation. Their principles are still relevant and were adopted by the National Health Service Breast Project in 1990 (Box 8.2 overleaf). In fact, these principles apply to all diseases, and many of them will be picked up in the case study of CHD later in this chapter.

Box 8.2 General principles of screening

1   The condition screened for should pose an important health problem.

2   The natural history of the condition should be well understood.

3   There should be a recognisable latent or early stage.

4   Treatment of the disease at an early stage should be of more benefit than treatment started at a later stage.

5   There should be a suitable test or examination.

6   The test or examination should be acceptable to the population.

7   For diseases of insidious onset, screening should be repeated at intervals determined by the natural history of the disease.

8   There should be adequate facilities available for the diagnosis and treatment of any abnormalities detected.

9   The chance of physical or psychological harm should be less than the chance of benefit.

10 The cost of case-finding (including diagnosis and subsequent treatment) should be economically balanced against the benefit it provides.

(Austoker, 1990, for the National Health Service Breast Project)

Principle 5 is stated in deceptively simple terms: we need to ask what criteria are used to judge whether a screening test is indeed 'suitable'? All such tests are evaluated to assess the extent to which they actually detect the disease or risk factor that they claim to measure. Two questions are important:

1   Is the test **sensitive**: does it detect *all* diseases/risk factors reliably?

2   Is the test **specific**: does it detect *only* the disease/risk factor being screened for?

A screening test that is insufficiently *sensitive* would result in **false negatives**, samples that are incorrectly recorded as 'normal', with potentially serious, sometimes life-threatening consequences from treatment delay. During the 1990s, confidence in the cervical screening programme in the NHS was affected when several hospitals detected an unacceptably high rate of false negatives among samples they had screened over a number of years. The consequences of a test that is inadequately *specific*, resulting in **false positives**, are also serious; the false result engenders considerable anxiety for the recipient who is then exposed to further testing to reveal the true picture. In both cases the health service must bear the significant extra cost of recalling and re-testing patients.

Sensitivity and specificity are not independent of one another; improving the sensitivity automatically makes a test less specific, and vice versa. There is thus a 'trade off' between the two. Furthermore, the effectiveness of screening is dependent upon being able to detect small changes in people who are not only uniquely variable, but most of whom do not have the disease or risk factor in question. It is not surprising, therefore, that screening inevitably produces some false-negative and false-positive results. The dilemma is in deciding where to draw the line between an 'acceptable' failure rate and inadequate practice.

8.3.2 Screening populations or individuals?

There are two main approaches to disease prevention through screening, which also affect its potential effectiveness.

In **population screening** (or **mass screening**) the whole of the population, or everyone in a particular group, for example an age-band, is investigated for the early signs of a specific disease or the presence of a risk factor. In 'named' screening, there is an intention to treat those individuals whose disease or risk factor is detected by the test, as in the example of newborn babies with PKU mentioned earlier. If they are detected early and put on a carefully controlled diet, the brain damage that would otherwise result can be prevented. Population screening can also be carried out 'anonymously' to determine the prevalence of that condition in the population. This has been the case, for example, in population screening for HIV, which is carried out anonymously on pregnant women in the UK during routine antenatal blood tests.

● Can anonymous screening of populations contribute to disease prevention?

■ It has no direct benefit for the people whose disease or risk factor is detected by the test, since no treatment or health education can be offered to them; but indirectly it may reduce the incidence of disease by informing better targeted health-education campaigns, and providing supporting evidence for health-protection legislation or for increased provision of curative services.

In **high-risk screening** (or **individual screening**), individuals who are thought to be at higher than average risk are screened selectively, often during routine consultation with health professionals, to establish whether early disease or a risk factor is indeed present. An example in the UK is the screening of individuals from certain ethnic groups that have a relatively high risk of certain genetically determined blood disorders such as thalassaemia, Tay-Sachs disease or sickle-cell disease.[3] Usually, the test is carried out only on family members when an affected baby is born, revealing the carrier status of its parents and raising concerns about preventing the birth of further affected children. This is also the case with cystic fibrosis, the commonest genetic disorder affecting white populations of European origin.

Although conditions such as these can be detected early and genetic counselling is generally offered to affected couples intending to have a family, no fully effective treatment is yet available. Where carriers of abnormal genes are identified, the only form of 'prevention' possible is to avoid reproduction, and where screening consists of pre-natal testing, termination of an affected pregnancy is the only 'preventive' option available. This example illustrates the difficult choices that may have to be made about the value of screening and points to the ethical dilemmas that inevitably emerge.

8.3.3 Ethics of screening

Principle 9 of the general principles of screening (Box 8.2) raises a major ethical dilemma for screening programmes in requiring that *the chance of physical or psychological harm should be less than the chance of benefit*. Where the outcome of a test is the decision to terminate an affected fetus, the assessment of benefit versus harm is the most difficult of all. Even where the issues being weighed in the balance directly affect only the patient, disease-prevention programmes based on screening

---

[3] A TV programme for OU students entitled 'Bloodlines – A family legacy' and an audiotape 'Tinkering with nature' explore issues raised by screening for and treating the blood disorders thalassaemia and haemophilia; they are associated with *Human Biology and Health: An Evolutionary Approach* (Open University Press, 3rd edn 2001). Genetic screening and its consequences are discussed in more detail in Chapters 4 and 9 of that book.

Table 8.2 Adverse psychological, social and ethical effects of disease-prevention programmes.

Adverse effect	Examples
Anticipated discomfort or perceived adverse effects	Pain from needle puncture for blood tests. Pain from breast compression during mammography. Fear of radiation from mammography. Unpleasantness of diet or exercise.
Unpleasant interactions with health-care workers	Unpleasantness of dealing with curt or uncommunicative personnel in a mammographic screening centre.
Time required	Guilt or anxiety concerning time taken from work or family. Decrease in functioning at work or at home.
Personal financial costs	Loss of income because of time taken from work. Payment for specific investigations or prescriptions.
Excessive overall awareness of health	Change in perception of general health resulting from worry over elevated cholesterol level or risk of heart disease, stroke or cancer.
Anxiety over the results of a screening test	Specific worry that the result of the screening test will be positive.
Implications of a positive result of a screening test	Anxiety over the consequences of having a specific disease. Decrease in social functioning because of anxiety and time required for further evaluation.
Being labelled as 'sick' or 'at high risk' because of a positive result of a screening test	Decrease in social functioning.
Psychopathological effects of preventive programmes	Eating disorder caused by dieting.
False assurance of disease-free status	False sense of security resulting from true-negative or false-negative test result.
Failure to obtain informed consent	Loss of autonomy. Lack of knowledge of possible adverse effects.

Source: Marshall, K. (1996) 'Prevention. How much harm? How much benefit?', *Canadian Medical Association Journal,* **155** (2), pp.169 – 76; also reproduced in The Open University (2001) K203 *Working for Health*, Block 3, Unit 14, Table 5, p. 156.

have the potential for physical as well as psychological harm, as indicated in Table 8.2.

Clearly, none of the possibilities outlined in Table 8.2 is inevitable, and certainly 'unpleasant' interactions with health-care workers ought not to happen. Other examples of these adverse effects will apply to some people and not others. For instance, those on low incomes or in occupations where it is difficult to get time off work will suffer greater adverse consequences than more affluent workers or those with more job control.

Genetic screening raises another set of ethical dilemmas, especially if there is no therapeutic advantage from acquiring the knowledge of one's own or one's children's genetic inheritance, to offset the anxiety caused by the information. Additionally, knowledge of genetic susceptibility can have harmful economic effects in terms of employment and insurance prospects. Screening and preventive interventions in general have been accused of interfering in people's lives. This falls into what David Armstrong (1995), a medical sociologist, calls 'surveillance medicine'. Screening techniques, particularly genetic screening, allow for the surveillance of our innermost being, and many people find this alarming. Linda McKie, a health psychologist, equates surveillance with control and in relation to cervical screening claims that the cervix:

> … is a site for state, professional and male surveillance and control, through a preventive service which many feel obligated to participate in. (McKie, 1995, p. 441)

The sense of obligation that McKie refers to raises another ethical dilemma. How free is the choice offered to individuals when failure to take a preventive measure results in a disease being contracted? Women who do not take up the chance for mammography or cervical screening services are often seen as feckless, or wilfully careless of their health. This issue is becoming more stark in relation to health-damaging behaviour, such as smoking; later in the chapter, we refer to the debate about whether persistent smokers have the right to expect medical treatment for 'self-inflicted' illness.

There is also an equity issue, because better-off people (who are generally at lower risk of developing most preventable diseases) are able to pay for health 'check ups' in the private sector, potentially benefiting from a range of screening tests.

At the turn of the new millennium the need to adopt effective disease-prevention strategies took on greater significance in the UK as a focus for government action. In England, the White Paper *Saving Lives: Our Healthier Nation* (Department of Health, 1999f) set four targets: to reduce deaths from heart disease and stroke, accidents and cancers, and to reduce the prevalence of poor mental health. CHD is high on the list of targets for reduction in mortality and morbidity, and so makes an excellent case study around which to tease out some of the dilemmas that we have discussed.

8.4 Preventing coronary heart disease: a case study

8.4.1 The scope of the CHD problem

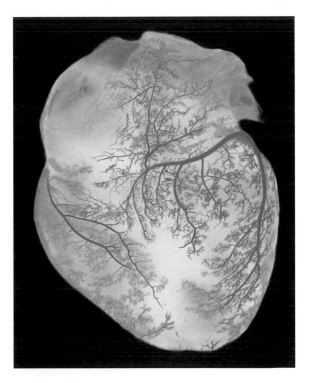

There are many different disease conditions or developmental abnormalities affecting the heart; in this chapter, we are focusing on the prevention of **coronary heart disease** (CHD). The condition is caused by an insufficient blood supply from the coronary arteries, which supply oxygen and nutrients to the heart muscle (myocardium), enabling it to sustain the rhythmic heart beat.

Narrowing within the coronary arteries is most commonly due to a build-up of fatty deposits called *plaques* on the inner wall of the artery, which eventually

The coronary arteries, which lie on (and crown) the outer wall of the heart, supply oxygenated blood to the heart muscle (myocardium), fuelling the action of the heart beat. There are three main coronary vessels, each with a fine tracery of capillaries branching outwards, which are clearly visible in this 'false coloured' image of a normal human heart. (Photo: Science Photo Library)

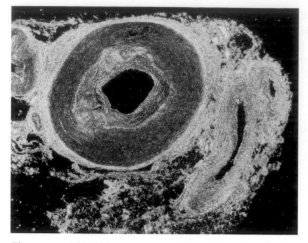

become hardened (a condition known as **atherosclerosis**). Such narrowing reduces the space available through which blood can flow and leads to a reduction in the amount of oxygen delivered to the heart muscle. (The medical term for restriction of oxygen supply is 'ischaemia', and medical texts often refer to *ischaemic heart disease* rather than coronary heart disease.) A person with atherosclerosis in one or more of their coronary arteries may experience **angina**, the chest 'tightness' brought on by exercise and relieved by rest.

The space within this coronary artery has been greatly reduced by hardened fatty deposits (plaques) on its inner wall, which restrict the amount of blood that can flow through it to supply the heart muscle. Plaques may also rupture or break off, blocking the circulation of blood to the heart completely and triggering a heart attack. (Photo: Eye of Science/Science Photo Library)

The plaques can also rupture and lead to clot (thrombus) formation, completely blocking or obstructing blood flow through the artery. This is the main cause of a heart attack or **myocardial infarction** (MI), in which the segment of heart muscle previously supplied by the coronary artery dies owing to lack of oxygen and nutrients.

In Chapter 6 you learned about the steps in a rational decision-making model, which can be applied to topics for health-care evaluation (Figure 6.1). Step 1 involves identifying and agreeing on the nature of the health problem. CHD is one of the most thoroughly investigated diseases because it is the most common cause of death in the UK, killing around 170 000 people a year by the end of the 1990s. Figure 8.1 shows that the majority of deaths occur after age 74, but CHD is also the main cause of 'premature' death in people below this age. Although the incidence (number of new cases per year) has been falling in the UK since the 1970s in people below age 74, in recent years it has been rising in the older age group.

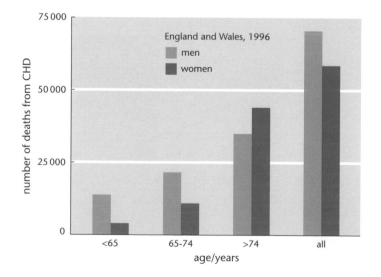

Figure 8.1 *Total number of deaths from coronary heart disease in men and women in different age groups, England and Wales, 1996. (Data derived from McPherson, K., Britton, A. and Causer, L., 2001,* Monitoring the progress of the 2010 target for coronary heart disease mortality: Estimated consequences on CHD incidence and mortality from changing prevalence of risk factors, *Table 1, p. 6, abstracted from the Office for National Statistics* Twentieth Century Mortality CD-ROM.)

● Figure 8.1 shows that, in 1996 in England and Wales, fewer women than men died from CHD below age 74, but that the position was reversed above age 74. What could explain this pattern?

■ One factor is that women on average live longer than men, and fewer men survive long enough to die from CHD beyond 74 years (remember that Figure 8.1 shows the total *number* of deaths in each age group). Also women seem to become more vulnerable to CHD after the menopause (a point to which we return below in the discussion of risk factors), so as they age CHD accounts for a greater proportion of female deaths.

In the UK it is estimated that around 300 000 people have a heart attack each year (Department of Health, 2000i). This is a sudden and frightening event and around half die before reaching hospital. Over a quarter of a million new cases of CHD are diagnosed in the UK each year, adding to the huge burden of morbidity from this condition; for example, 1.4 million people suffer from angina, and a million from some form of heart failure. Given these statistics, it is not surprising that CHD has provoked a lot of anxiety and calls for effective action at all levels, either to prevent its occurrence or at least to reduce the number of deaths and the extent of morbidity.

However, intervening in the complex degenerative processes that eventually lead to CHD is far from straightforward. One of the most pressing problems is in determining the nature and relative importance of the many potential risk factors, and unravelling how they interact with an individual's biology to produce damage in the coronary arteries and heart muscle.

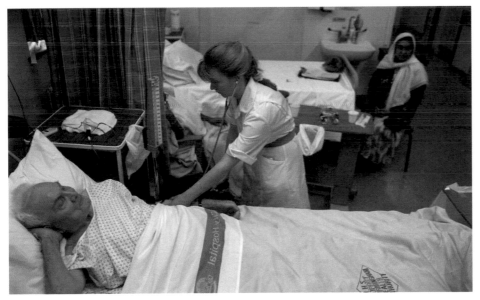

A staff nurse takes a patient's blood pressure in a coronary care unit, the main site of treatment following a myocardial infarction (heart attack). (Photo: John Harris/Report Digital)

8.4.2 Who is at risk of CHD?

International comparisons

A major source of evidence on risk factors for CHD comes from international comparisons of disease rates in different countries. Figure 8.2 (*overleaf*) presents some of the results from a project set up by the World Health Organisation (WHO) to monitor trends and investigate the risk factors for CHD in 38 populations in 21 countries over a 10-year period, from the mid-1980s to the mid-1990s. This huge research study – known as the WHO MONICA Project (MONItoring trends and determinants in CArdiovascular disease) – recorded, among other data, the combined total of all coronary deaths and non-fatal heart attacks (the 'coronary event rate' in Figure 8.2). All the CHD rates have been standardised for age against

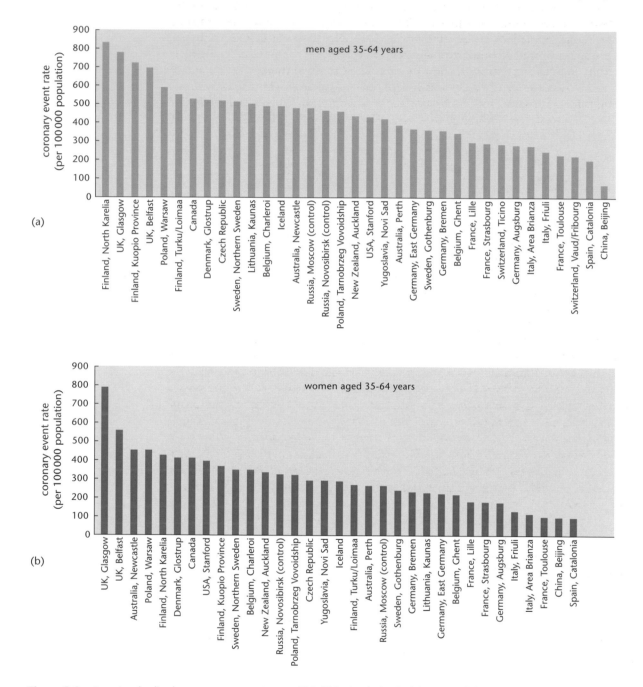

(a)

(b)

Figure 8.2 *Age-standardised coronary event rates per 100 000 population in (a) men and (b) women aged 35–64, in the World Health Organisation's 38 MONICA Project populations, latest data available in 2000. This project monitors international trends and determinants in cardiovascular disease. (Source: Petersen, S., Rayner, M, and Press, V., 2000, Coronary Heart Disease Statistics: 2000 edition, British Heart Foundation Health Promotion Research Group, University of Oxford, Figures 2.1a and b, p. 43)*

the European standard population; age-standardisation means that rates can be compared over time and among countries despite differences in the age structure of their populations.[4]

● Briefly summarise what seem to you to be the most striking features of Figure 8.2.

■ The first point you probably noticed was the high coronary event rate in the two UK populations (Glasgow and Belfast) for both men and women, relative to other populations around the world. Secondly, these data confirm that in the age group 35–64 the coronary event rate is higher in men than in women from the same population, and in most locations the male rate is roughly twice that of females. Glasgow is exceptional in having similar coronary event rates for both sexes and the highest rate for women of any population in the study, with women from Belfast in second place.

● What grounds for optimism can be drawn from Figure 8.2 that the depressingly high CHD rates in the UK could be reduced by appropriate disease prevention strategies? Why might this be difficult to achieve?

■ The fact that most populations have CHD rates so much lower than those in the UK – generally less than half the UK rates and at best below a quarter (e.g. compare Catalonia in Spain with Glasgow and Belfast) – strongly suggests that CHD can be reduced in the UK. The difficulty is in determining what features of the 'low risk' populations could be transferred to the 'high risk' populations with similarly beneficial effects.

Another encouraging sign is that three indicators – the incidence of new cases of CHD in people below 74, the overall mortality rate, and the *case-fatality rate* (the proportion of people with CHD who die) – have all been falling in the UK since the 1970s, in common with the trend in most industrialised countries around the world. However, as a consequence, *morbidity* rates are rising, because people who would previously have died are now living with symptoms such as angina and breathlessness. A study published in 2001 reported that the rates of CHD diagnosed among adult men in Britain had not fallen in the previous 20 years, even though their death rates had gone down (Lampe *et al.*, 2001). In 1998, just over 15 per cent of men and 10 per cent of women living in Britain in the age group 45–64 reported symptoms of premature heart disease such as chest pain; the proportions affected rose to 28 per cent of men and 27 per cent of women aged 65–74, and 31 per cent and 30 per cent, respectively, at age 75 and above (ONS, 2000b). A further sobering thought is that CHD mortality rates are rising in *developing* countries, where the challenges for disease-prevention strategies are far greater than in the UK.[5]

Variations in CHD risk between groups in the UK

International comparisons such as the MONICA Project reveal variations in CHD risk between countries, but there are equally striking variations between different groups in the *same* country. In the UK, the most striking 'inequalities' in the

[4] The importance of age-standardisation is described and illustrated in *Studying Health and Disease* (Open University Press, 2nd edn 1994; colour-enhanced 2nd edn 2001), Chapter 7, and in *World Health and Disease* (Open University Press, 3rd edn 2001), Chapter 2.

[5] The so-called 'epidemiological transition' in developing countries, which occurs as mortality from communicable diseases declines and deaths from chronic degenerative diseases increase, is discussed in *World Health and Disease* (Open University Press, 3rd edn 2001), Chapters 6 and 8.

distribution of CHD occur between the sexes, between members of different social classes (as defined by the Registrar General's classification on the basis of occupation of head of household[6]), and between different ethnic groups. Research into the underlying determinants of these patterns has shed considerable light on the causal factors contributing to CHD, and thus points the way towards preventive actions.

Figures 8.1 and 8.2 have already illustrated the relatively greater risk of CHD experienced by men compared with women from the same age-group and population. This sexual division in CHD is poorly understood. One explanation is that oestrogen may offer some protection against CHD, since the incidence in women increases after the menopause, but the evidence for an oestrogen effect is inconclusive. Initial reports showed reductions in CHD in post-menopausal women taking hormone replacement therapy (HRT), but later studies have generally not provided sufficient evidence of CHD prevention to justify the small increase in risk of certain cancers. In 2001 the American Medical Association issued a statement advising against the prescription of HRT primarily as a preventive measure against heart disease.

A study of long-term trends in mortality from CHD cast further doubt on the assumption that the lower rates in women are due to protection from oestrogen. Lawlor, Ebrahim and Davey Smith (2001) plotted death rates in England and Wales for men and women between 1921 and 1998, and found that the 'twentieth century epidemic' of CHD had affected only men from the 1940s onwards. The rates of CHD among women remained virtually unchanged while men's rates soared until they reached their peak in the 1970s. Similar patterns were found for men and women in other industrialised countries.

● How does this finding undermine the idea that oestrogen protects women from CHD?

■ If this were true, you would have to postulate that women produced higher and higher levels of oestrogen from the 1940s to the 1970s, thereby counteracting whatever environmental factors were driving up the CHD rates in men.

It must be stressed that this study does not show that biological differences between men and women have *no* impact on their divergent CHD rates. But it strongly suggests that rather than thinking of women's rates as being 'reduced' by their biology, we should instead see men's rates as being 'elevated' by their greater exposure to factors that promote CHD.

There is persuasive evidence that the different patterns of exposure, lifestyles and social worlds inhabited by men and women also contribute to their relative risks of CHD. Thus disease-prevention strategies aimed at reducing male deaths from CHD to female levels may need to address *gender* differences rather than *sex* differences. For example, men are less likely than women to consult a doctor when they feel ill, at least partly because they are more likely to be in full-time jobs where taking time off is difficult. Men and women may have different patterns of fat consumption, or different responses to dietary fat. Whatever the explanation, the importance of social factors in the aetiology of CHD is unequivocally demonstrated by research on social class.

[6] The use of the Registrar General's classification to distinguish social class groups raises several technical issues that have to be considered when interpreting the results of epidemiological and social surveys; these are discussed in *World Health and Disease* (Open University Press, 3rd edn 2001), Chapters 9 and 10, which also analyses data on the social class gradient in health in the UK.

Inequalities in health have gradually moved up the health-policy agenda in the UK since the publication of the Black Report (DHSS, London, 1980). The **social class gradient in CHD** is one of the most striking examples: men from the semi-skilled and unskilled manual classes IV and V are three times more likely to die prematurely from CHD than those in the managerial and professional classes I and II. If the death rate in all manual classes combined is compared with the rate in all non-manual classes for each sex (Figure 8.3), it becomes apparent that despite the overall falling trend in mortality from CHD, the gap between these two social class groupings has become steadily wider over time in men. In women, the gap was closing up to the mid-1980s, but then began to widen again.

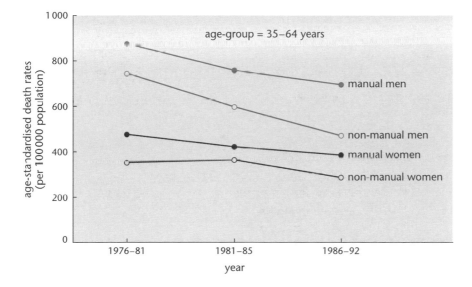

Figure 8.3 *Trends in age-standardised CHD mortality rates per 100 000 population in men and women aged 35–64 years from manual and non-manual social classes in England and Wales, 1976–1992. (Data derived from Drever, F. and Whitehead, M., 1997,* Health Inequalities: Decennial Supplement, *DS series no. 15, The Stationery Office, London, Tables 11.5 and 11.7, using the Registrar General's social classification on the basis of occupation of head of household.)*

In the UK, the most influential research on the determinants of the social class gradient in CHD has come from the longitudinal Whitehall I and II studies, which began in 1967, and track the health of two cohorts of civil servants with a combined total of almost 30 000 people. The results have confirmed a *gradient* in the risk of CHD in men and women in 'white collar' occupations, with those in the most senior grades experiencing the lowest CHD rates, those in the next grade down experiencing higher CHD rates, and so on down the gradient, to the worst CHD rates in those in the lowest employment grades (for example, see Marmot *et al.*, 2001).

The Whitehall studies have also provided powerful evidence of various risk factors that contribute to the unequal distribution of CHD in the population, and which have also been demonstrated in many other countries. You probably know about the so-called **classical risk factors for CHD** from health-education campaigns.

● Can you list them?

■ They are raised levels of cholesterol in the blood, smoking, raised blood pressure (hypertension), physical inactivity and obesity.

Their contribution to the risk of developing CHD is discussed below, when we consider primary prevention strategies aimed at changing the level of risk. The Whitehall II study has uniquely established that even when the effects of these classical risk factors have been excluded, a social class gradient in CHD remains. Analyses of the possible explanations for this 'non-classical' risk points to features of the work that people do and its effects on their self-esteem – CHD is more common in employment grades where the workers have low control over their job, experience greater monotony and use fewer skills (Bosma *et al.*, 1997). There is also evidence that other psychosocial factors can adversely affect health, as Chapter 9 will describe.

● Can you think of other possible contributors to the social gradient in CHD?

■ Difficulties with accessing health and social services, or relevant sources of information (including on the Internet), may restrict the ability of people on low incomes to prevent disease, or reduce its impact, in themselves and their families. For example, they may find it harder to get to a GP surgery, and may not have seen health-education messages about CHD risk factors, or realise that they can ask for a screening test.

Ethnic differences are also apparent in the distribution of CHD within the UK population. For example, among people living in the UK who were born in the Indian sub-continent, the death rate from CHD is 38 per cent higher for men and 43 per cent higher for women than rates for England and Wales as a whole (Wild and McKeigue, 1997). The debate among researchers continues about whether these differences in disease risk are cultural, socio-economic or biological in origin, but low access to health information and health services is clearly a factor.

Although ethnicity is strongly linked with risk for CHD, migrant studies show that the link between ethnicity and CHD is not fixed. For example, Japanese people living in Japan have a very low risk of CHD, but Japanese migrants to the USA quickly develop risk levels similar to the host population. This suggests that explanations at the level of biological vulnerability to CHD are inadequate.

● How might the factors described above interact in ways that increase the risk of developing CHD?

■ The highest risks are likely to be experienced by men who smoke and are overweight, working in monotonous manual jobs that allow them minimal scope for autonomy and skill; such jobs are among the lowest paid, so stress generated from within the workplace is compounded by living on a low income; people from ethnic minorities are over-represented in such employment; a combination of stress, low self-esteem and low income make it more likely that the classical risk factors, such as smoking and obesity, will also be present.

Individual risk factors for CHD

What is clear from extensive research into the causes of CHD is that there is a complex relationship between the classical risk factors associated with this disease. 'Blame' cannot be apportioned between risk factors at the level of each individual who develops heart disease, but estimates of their relative contribution at the population level have been made by aggregating data from large-scale research, such as the MONICA Project and the Whitehall studies.

Figure 8.4 represents an estimation of how much each of the classical risk factors contributes to death rates from CHD in the UK in people under the age of 75. The total adds up to more than 100 per cent because the risk factors overlap, as shown in the diagram; thus a person who has both a high cholesterol level and high blood pressure counts more than once in the total — in this example, 59 per cent (46 + 13) of all cases of CHD are attributable to a combination of these two risk factors. [Note: the amount of cholesterol in the blood is measured in millimoles per

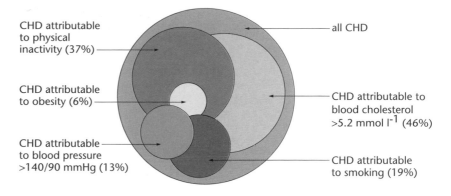

Figure 8.4 *Proportion of all CHD in the UK attributable to each of the classical risk factors in people under 75, both sexes combined. (Source: McPherson, K., Britton, A. and Causer, L., 2001,* Monitoring the progress of the 2010 target for coronary heart disease mortality: Estimated consequences on CHD incidence and mortality from changing prevalence of risk factors, *Appendix 2, p. 69, data abstracted from Petersen, S., Rayner, M. and Press, V., 2000,* Coronary Heart Disease Statistics: 2000 edition, *British Heart Foundation Health Promotion Group, University of Oxford.)*

litre, which is written on Figure 8.4 in scientific notation as $mmol\,l^{-1}$; blood pressure is measured as the height in millimetres (mm) of a column of mercury (chemical symbol, Hg) sustained in a gauge, and is recorded first when the heart contracts (e.g. 140 mmHg) and then when it relaxes (e.g. 90 mmHg).]

The largest proportion of CHD (46 per cent in Figure 8.4) is attributed to raised cholesterol in the blood, but estimating the risk for an *individual* is not straightforward. People with the highest cholesterol levels (above $8\,mmol\,l^{-1}$) certainly have the highest coronary risk, but as Figure 8.5 shows, only a very small proportion of the population fall into this category. Below this level it is much more difficult to evaluate individual risk because the difference between what is considered to be a 'normal' cholesterol level and what is 'very high' is relatively small. A cholesterol level of $5.2\,mmol\,l^{-1}$

is taken to be on the borderline of normal, whereas $8\,mmol\,l^{-1}$ would be considered dangerously high. Figure 8.5 shows that cholesterol levels in men who went on to develop CHD are not much higher than in men who did not, and it illustrates a further major problem – the two curves overlap considerably. It is therefore impossible to tell whether a man with a raised cholesterol level of (for example) $6.5\,mmol\,l^{-1}$ is going to develop CHD.

The uncertainty is partly because blood cholesterol is found in two forms,

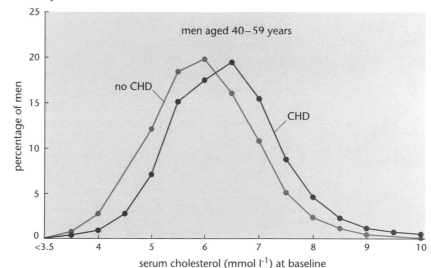

Figure 8.5 *Blood cholesterol levels in British men aged 40–59, showing those who went on to develop CHD and those who did not. (Source: Ebrahim, S., Davey Smith, G., McCabe, C. et al., 1998, Cholesterol and coronary heart disease: screening and treatment, Quality in Health Care, 7, Figure 2, p. 233.)*

low-density lipoprotein (or LDL–cholesterol), which is considered to be harmful, and high-density lipoprotein (or HDL–cholesterol), which is not. The ratio between the two is a better but not absolute measure of CHD risk.

A similar problem is evident when trying to apply to individuals the population risk of CHD that is attributed to raised blood pressure (13 per cent in Figure 8.4). In the UK an estimated 41 per cent of adult men and 33 per cent of adult women have hypertension, and clearly they don't all develop CHD. Moreover, observing an association between CHD and raised blood pressure does not prove causality.

● What other explanation can you suggest?

■ It could be that raised blood pressure is a product of CHD, rather than a cause.

Physical inactivity is another major risk factor for CHD, contributing to 37 per cent of the total according to Figure 8.4. Weight gain is also thought to be due in part to a lack of exercise. One type of obesity has been specifically linked to CHD, the accumulation of fat in the abdomen rather than the thighs and arms – a distribution known as **central obesity**. It is estimated by measuring the waist-to-hip ratio, and the higher this ratio the higher the risk of CHD.

One firmly established risk for CHD is that of smoking, where a clear association has been shown with the number of cigarettes smoked per day and with the number of years as a smoker (McPherson et al., 2001, Table 20). Carbon monoxide in tobacco smoke is absorbed into the bloodstream and displaces some of the oxygen that normally would have reached the heart. This makes the heart work harder and faster. The effect of the key component of nicotine in cigarettes also acts on the blood by reducing its capacity to deliver oxygen. The combined action of carbon monoxide and nicotine promotes atherosclerosis and causes coronary artery spasms and irregular heart rhythms. As well as its direct effects, smoking is also thought to promote CHD indirectly by increasing the ratio of LDL–cholesterol to HDL–cholesterol and raising blood pressure.

Since the mid-1970s there has been an overall decline in smoking in England, so that both the number of people who smoke and the number of cigarettes smoked have fallen. When smokers quit, their risk of CHD attributable to smoking declines and at least part of the downward population trend in CHD is due to the reduction in smoking. There are, however, important variations in smoking rates between groups, which are thought to explain, at least in part, the unequal distribution of CHD described earlier. For example, although men were formerly much more likely to smoke than women, since about 1980 this gap has narrowed, and the rate of uptake in younger people has increased, particularly among girls. There are regional differences too, most prominently the rates of smoking are higher in Scotland and Northern Ireland than in England and Wales. And there is a higher incidence of smoking in manual than in non-manual social classes. Finally, smoking rates vary between ethnic groups, with the highest rates in Bangladeshi men and Caribbean men and women (Department of Health, 2000j).

The interaction of smoking with so many other classical risk factors, and with social, regional and ethnic dimensions, illustrates why it is impossible to generate accurate risk assessments for individuals. This uncertainty creates dilemmas for any attempts to prevent CHD. Prevention is particularly problematic because the disease involves a complex degenerative process, which develops over the life course and in which many causal and contributory factors are involved.

8.4.3 Dilemmas in CHD prevention

Primary prevention

Primary prevention relies on intervening effectively before the disease process begins. Given the high prevalence of CHD, you could conclude either that we are *all* at risk or that it is impossible to determine accurately who is at risk, and therefore some form of mass intervention that reaches the whole population would be most effective.

● What strategies have you encountered that aim to reduce the incidence of CHD in the population?

■ You have probably seen posters advising you to 'look after your heart' by giving up smoking, eating a low-fat diet with plenty of fresh fruit and vegetables, losing weight if you are overweight for your height, moderating your alcohol intake, and participating regularly in strenuous exercise.

The problem with mass health-education campaigns is that they are not very effective at persuading people to change their behaviour. One reason for this is that it is difficult for most of us to feel motivated enough to alter our lifestyle when the threat to our health seems a long way off. Because most people *don't* develop CHD, how can an individual assess whether making behavioural changes now would actually bring any health gain later in life?

Another problem is that the reductions in CHD that are likely to flow from acting on advice about changes in lifestyle are relatively modest, and campaigns cannot claim that behavioural change will guarantee protection from CHD. For example, it has been estimated that the incidence of new cases of CHD could be reduced by 9 per cent by 2010 if everyone whose physical activity is currently light or sedentary could increase it to a 'moderate' level, i.e. three sessions per week of moderate exercise lasting 20 minutes (McPherson *et al.,* 2001). This study also estimated that lowering cholesterol levels could reduce CHD incidence by 10 per cent over the same period. If everyone in England followed *all* the advice on lifestyle changes, then a possible 30 per cent reduction in new cases of CHD is considered feasible by 2010 – resulting in 78 000 fewer new cases per year than at the turn of the millennium. But how likely is it that such widespread behavioural changes will occur?

● Suggest some of the reasons why behavioural change is difficult to achieve.

■ The material circumstances of people's lives can erect powerful barriers to change; for example, low-income families may be unable to afford the recommended 'healthy' diet, join a gym or pay entrance fees to the swimming pool; low-paid jobs are the most likely to have unsocial hours with short breaks, forcing workers to eat snack meals and restricting leisure time for sports activity; people whose lives are stressed by insecurity or monotonous unskilled employment are most likely to use tobacco and alcohol to help them to cope.

On the basis of this analysis, tackling CHD effectively will require far-reaching structural and economic changes in society. An obvious dilemma in such a massive programme would be how to fund it, whether from cuts in public services, increases in taxation, or borrowing huge sums and increasing the national debt (a topic to which we return in Chapter 9).

The alternative strategy to mass prevention campaigns is to target individuals who are considered to be most at risk. At the local level, interventions might involve an initiative such as a health authority setting up 'quit smoking' classes, or a GP deciding to measure the waist-to-hip ratio of every adult who appears to be overweight, and giving advice on dietary change. The drawback about such *ad hoc* activity is that it is hard to administer and evaluate systematically.

In an attempt to address this problem, national guidelines for tackling CHD were published by the Department of Health in 2000 in a National Service Framework (NSF) on CHD. It set 12 'standards' for reducing the burden of heart disease in the population, three of which relate to primary prevention:

> The NHS and partner agencies should
>
> - develop, implement and monitor policies that reduce the prevalence of coronary risk factors in the population, and reduce inequalities in risks of developing heart disease;
>
> - contribute to a reduction in the prevalence of smoking in the local population.
>
> General practitioners and primary care teams should
>
> - identify all people at significant risk of cardiovascular disease but who have not developed symptoms and offer them appropriate advice and treatment to reduce their risks. (Department of Health, 2000i, p.14)

The other nine standards relate to secondary prevention and focus on the early detection and effective care of people with suspected or proven heart disease, with the aim of reducing morbidity and mortality. The CHD National Service Framework gives details of the actions that should be taken by the various agencies and health professionals by certain dates. The Department of Health's target is to reduce deaths from circulatory diseases (of which CHD is the most prevalent), saving up to 200 000 lives in total in England by 2010, i.e. ten years after publication of the NSF. This would represent a fall in mortality of about 40 per cent. Even higher targets have been set in separate national guidelines for Scotland and Northern Ireland, where CHD rates are higher than in the rest of the UK (Scottish Office, 1999; DHSS, Belfast, 1997).

These are laudable aims, but GPs were quick to see that the lion's share of the work in implementing the NSF's primary-prevention strategies would fall on them and their practice staff. A study of the implications for general practice workloads concluded that, in an average practice serving 10 000 patients, 2 221 disease-control measures would be needed annually to meet the NSF's guidelines, and a total of 904 entries would have to be made in patients' computer records (Hippisley-Cox and Pringle, 2001).

● Aside from the strain on primary-care staff from this increased workload, what potential drawbacks might it have for patients?

■ Meeting the NSF targets is very likely to incur an 'opportunity cost' (Chapter 2) in that the resources required are so substantial that they will divert some health-care activity from other services for patients.

Historically, the resources devoted to the primary prevention of CHD have been small relative to other health-care and social-care expenditure on existing CHD patients, as Figure 8.6 shows. The government have pledged additional funds to support the NSF targets, but there is doubt about whether it will meet the costs of the extra workload involved.

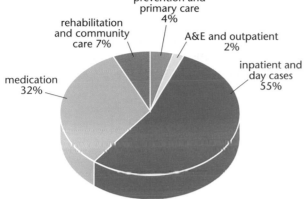

Figure 8.6 *Distribution of the costs of CHD to the NHS and the social-care system in the UK in 1996. (Source: Petersen, S., Rayner, M. and Press, V., 2000, Coronary Heart Disease Statistics: 2000 edition, British Heart Foundation Health Promotion Research Group, University of Oxford, Figure 13.1, p. 130.) (A&E: Accident and Emergency departments)*

Nevertheless, you might argue that preventing CHD should be given a very high priority, if 200 000 lives could indeed be saved by 2010. However, the 'gold standard' of evidence (as discussed in Chapter 6) suggests that this target is unlikely to be reached; a Cochrane Collaboration Systematic Review of 18 clinical trials concluded that:

> The pooled effects suggest multiple risk factor intervention has no effect on mortality ... however, a small but potentially important benefit, up to 10 per cent relative reduction in CHD mortality reduction may have been missed. (Ebrahim and Davey Smith, 2001)

The authors also commented that the intensive interventions used in many clinical trials 'far exceed what is feasible in routine practice'. This evaluation takes us to the central dilemma in the prevention of CHD, as expressed in an editorial in the *British Medical Journal*:

> Is it ethical to encourage primary care to divert resources into primary prevention screening and interventions with such modest benefits? (Toop and Richards, 2001, p. 247)

Health education aimed at primary prevention of CHD is also beginning to make an appearance in antenatal clinics, as a result of the wide publicity given to the *fetal programming hypothesis* developed by David Barker and colleagues (reviewed in O'Brien, Wheeler and Barker, 1999).[7] The evidence remains controversial but suggests that undernutrition of the fetus and slow growth in infancy may lead to irreversible changes in the structure of the baby's developing blood vessels, which in turn increase the susceptibility to CHD (among other conditions) in later life. Poor diet and smoking during pregnancy have thus become even greater targets for change by concerned health professionals, but this raises the dilemma that attendance at antenatal clinics could fall if mothers feel 'accused' of inflicting lifelong damage on their offspring.

---

[7] The research studies on which the fetal programming hypothesis is based are described in *Studying Health and Disease* (Open University Press, 2nd edn 1994; colour-enhanced 2nd edn 2001), Chapter 10, and in an audiotape for Open University students entitled 'Data interpretation: the programming hypothesis'.

Secondary prevention

Concerns about the workload implications of the CHD National Service Framework apply equally to secondary prevention, both in terms of hospital procedures and primary care for people living with the disease.

Perhaps the most contentious issue has been the target set for high-risk screening, which requires GPs to identify and treat individuals whose risk factors are above certain limits. This raises the dilemma of where to draw the line between 'normal' and 'high risk', and between 'treatment' and 'no treatment'. Large numbers of people with moderate risk factors could be missed if the line is drawn in the wrong place, yet these are the group in whom most cases occur. Targeted screening by GPs will have most success at intervening in the disease processes of the most vulnerable people with the highest risk factors, but the majority of the national disease burden from CHD does not occur at this end of the spectrum.

However, another dilemma in placing responsibility on GPs to identify high-risk individuals is that the people who are least likely to be registered with a GP, or attend the surgery for screening tests, are those whose social circumstances also place them at greatest risk of heart disease. How could they be reached?

● A mass screening programme that aimed to reach everyone would overcome this problem, but it raises ethical dilemmas. Can you suggest what they are?

■ The first is whether it is ethically acceptable to compel everyone to undertake screening tests that will inevitably result in some individuals being labelled as 'at increased risk' of CHD, but who will *not* go on to develop the disease (as Figure 8.5 showed). For these people, the psychological harm arising from screening outweighs the benefits (contravening principle 9 in Box 8.2). The second dilemma is whether everyone whose risk factors are above some notional level should be assisted in reducing them; the majority of these individuals would be altering their lifestyles 'unnecessarily', but collectively their actions would help to prevent CHD deaths in the rest.

One of the difficulties in establishing a secondary prevention programme for people who already have CHD is that not everyone experiences warning symptoms, such as angina. Without such symptoms the only secure way to detect and diagnose narrowed coronary arteries 'early' is to perform an exploratory imaging test called an *angiogram*. A radio-opaque dye is injected into the coronary arteries so that the vessels show up on an X-ray film or imaging screen; blockages are identified when the dye cannot penetrate easily beyond a constriction point. However, it may be difficult to see on an angiogram what is going on beyond the constriction.

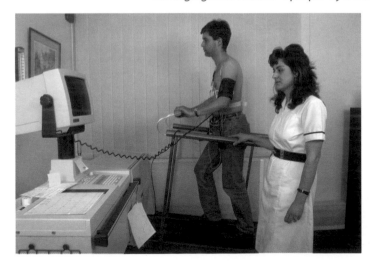

A technician in a hospital cardiology clinic conducts a 'stress test'. This patient who has symptoms of angina is walking on a treadmill and continuous electrocardiogram (ECG) monitoring is in progress, with the aim of capturing any changes from an angina episode on the tracing. (Photo: John Callan/Shout Picture Library)

Advances in MRI scanning (as discussed in Chapter 7) have made it possible to reveal the extent of narrowing within blood vessels, which can extend throughout their length. But there is much competition for MRI scans for other conditions (e.g. cancers) and it is a very expensive technology. Here again we encounter the dilemma of whether this is the 'best' use of scarce resources in terms of achieving the greatest benefit for the largest number, while incurring the least harm.

Another example of this dilemma occurs as a result of advances in treatment for high levels of cholesterol. Effective cholesterol-lowering drugs, called statins, can reduce the level in the minority of individuals in whom it is considered to be dangerously high. Such treatment has shown substantial reductions in heart attacks in this group of patients, but the cost to the NHS has been huge since these drugs became available – £93 million by 1996 in England alone, and rising (Petersen *et al.*, 2000, Table 2.3).

The fact that statins appear to benefit the highest-risk patients makes it harder to justify *not* prescribing them for people whose cholesterol level is a little below 'dangerously high', so the cut-off point creeps down and the cost spirals upwards. But audits have shown that as many as 80 per cent of people who might benefit from taking statins are not doing so (Primatesta and Poulter, 2000), which suggests that some form of rationing may be occurring. However, if statins were prescribed as recommended in the NSF, the cost to the NHS is estimated to rise to £1.5 *billion* per year (Petersen *et al.*, 2000). Also, these drugs are not without risk – a widely prescribed statin was withdrawn in the USA in 2001 when it was implicated in 31 deaths – so doctors may 'underuse' statins when faced with the dilemma of balancing potential benefits against potential harm.

Sex discrimination in the provision of secondary-prevention measures, including the prescription of statins, has also been reported in general practice (Hippisley-Cox, Pringle, Crown, Meal and Wynn, 2001). Women with a diagnosis of CHD were less likely than men to have had all their classical risk factors measured, or to have been prescribed cholesterol-lowering drugs, despite the fact that a higher proportion of women have raised blood cholesterol compared with men of the same age and social class.

The discussion of secondary prevention can be summed up in the following questions for which there are no straightforward answers. Is it possible to develop an effective and affordable approach to the reduction of CHD in high-risk individuals when there are so many interacting determinants of heart disease, and so many other calls on health-service resources? How can such a strategy target high-risk groups without appearing to 'blame the victims' for their illness? On an ethical level, can we expect people to change long-standing behaviour in order to reduce their CHD risks, when the evidence about what benefits might accrue is at best equivocal? Should behavioural change be aggressively promoted on the grounds that it will save lives, when this can also reduce individual autonomy and self-esteem, and compromise the right to choose one's own lifestyle?

Next we consider the overlapping domains of tertiary prevention and treatment for established CHD.

CABG and dilemmas in tertiary prevention

Of the many medical interventions that may reduce the effects or at least slow the progression of CHD, we have chosen to focus on the dilemmas arising from **coronary artery bypass grafting**, commonly known by the acronym CABG ('cabbage'). This procedure is prescribed for patients with severe atherosclerosis, which narrows

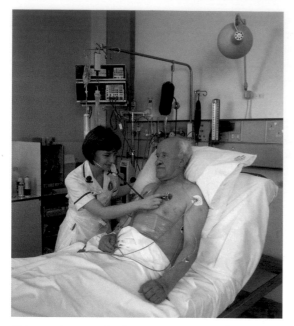

This man is recovering from coronary artery bypass grafting (CABG) in an intensive therapy unit (ITU). The number of people receiving this treatment doubled in the 1990s, putting increasing pressure on ITU provision; lack of an available ITU bed is a common reason for the postponement of operations.
(Photo: St Bartholomew's Hospital/Science Photo Library)

(occludes) one or more of the three main coronary arteries, with or without angina. It involves major surgery in which the blocked artery is bypassed using a grafted section of blood vessel taken from the patient's chest wall or leg. The number of people treated annually by CABG more than doubled between 1990 and 2000, and over 28 000 operations were carried out in 2000 in the UK (Petersen *et al.*, 2000).

The key dilemma in making this treatment decision is how a doctor is to determine which patients are appropriate for CABG. This involves judgement that the operation for a given patient will do more good than harm (the exact equivalent of principle 9 for screening, Box 8.2). However, doctors cannot turn to randomised controlled trials (RCTs) for evidence; RCTs will never be able to answer this question for the majority of patients because each patient presents a unique clinical picture. Moreover, trials to date (2001) have either been too small to answer questions about survival, or are too old to reflect how technology has moved on, or they have not recruited a representative sample of patients (a point we return to shortly).

An alternative method, developed by the RAND Corporation in the USA, involves a panel of experts formalising their judgement of appropriateness for CABG for a comprehensive list of patient scenarios. Each patient scenario comprises a unique combination of the severity of the angina, the number of diseased coronary arteries, the operative risk and so on. The outcomes of this exercise are central to the Appropriateness of Coronary Revascularisation (ACRE) study; one of its research findings is the subject of Figure 8.7.

Among patients in whom CABG is deemed appropriate following angiography, it is actually quite common for them to receive solely medical management; Figure 8.7 shows that these patients had a much higher probability of death or non-fatal heart attack than other 'appropriate' patients who underwent CABG. This suggests that CABG may be underused, and calls into question the decision-making process

Figure 8.7 *Mortality in 1 353 patients rated by an expert panel as appropriate for coronary artery bypass surgery (CABG), comparing those who did not get surgery with those who were treated medically. (Data from the ACRE study, Appropriateness of Coronary Revascularisation; the difference between groups was statistically significant (P < 0.001). Source: Hemingway, H. et al., 2001, Underuse of coronary revascularization procedures in patients considered appropriate candidates for revascularization, New England Journal of Medicine, **344**, Figure 1, p. 652. Copyright © 2001 Massachusetts Medical Society. All rights reserved.)*

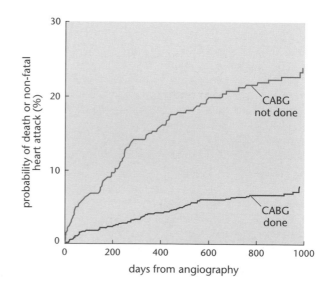

for surgical interventions. It is universally observed that individual clinicians vary widely in their decision-making; thus the same patient presenting to different doctors may be offered markedly different treatments. The ACRE study raises the dilemma as to whether the formalised recommendations of an expert panel based on 'scenario' patients may produce better outcomes than the variable decisions of individual clinicians faced with 'real' patients.

Another serious concern is about the evaluation of CABG. If you look back at Chapter 2, you will see from Table 2.1 that the largest cost-per-QALY gained from CABG follows treating those patients with the most severe coronary artery disease. Results such as these have focused attention on the need to prioritise waiting lists on the premise that those with the most severe symptoms or worst prognosis have the most to gain from earlier CABG.

● If the patients with the most severe symptoms are more likely to be selected for treatment, what impact do you think this has upon the evaluation of the *efficacy* of CABG?

■ You would expect there to be a *higher* mortality rate if the worst cases are given priority, because these are the patients who will be at greatest risk and who are, therefore, more likely to die than people with less severe coronary artery damage. Such prioritisation is therefore likely to bias the evaluation of efficacy.

Furthermore, there is evidence that studies of the relative merits of different treatments for CHD, including CABG, have been biased by the exclusion of patients in older age groups from intervention trials.

● This sort of age bias in research into CHD was first mentioned in Chapter 2. What justification is made for it and what effect might it have on the validity of the results?

■ Older people may be excluded on the grounds that they generally suffer from other degenerative conditions in addition to CHD; including them in trials of treatment therefore makes the results harder to interpret. But because the rates of CHD increase with age, excluding older people from trials means that treatments have largely been inadequately evaluated in the age group in which the disease is most prevalent.

'Ageism' among doctors is an alternative explanation and may partly underlie the lower rates at which older patients with CHD are referred for investigations and specialist treatments such as CABG (Bowling, 1999)[8].

An individual can do nothing to change his or her age – a statement that takes on a new resonance in the light of another highly controversial dilemma – whether interventions such as CABG should be offered to people who cannot or will not change their behaviour to improve their chances of a successful outcome. Both sides of the debate were published in the *British Medical Journal* in 1993; Open University students should now read the article in *Health and Disease: A Reader*

[8] An article by Ann Bowling, 'Ageism in cardiology', appears in *Health and Disease: A Reader* (Open University Press, 3rd edn 2001). It was optional reading for Open University students during an earlier book in this series, *Birth to Old Age: Health in Transition* (Open University Press, 2nd edn 1995; colour-enhanced 2nd edn 2001), Chapter 11; you should read it now, if you have not already done so.

(Open University Press, 3rd edn 2001) entitled 'Should smokers be offered coronary bypass surgery?' The arguments against are put by a researcher M. J. Underwood and a cardiac surgeon J. S. Bailey; then read the countervailing case put by Matthew Shiu, a GP.

● What dilemmas are raised by Underwood and Bailey?

■ They note that smoking has contributed to the damage in the coronary arteries, and it will have the same effect on the graft; this helps to explain why smokers are much more likely to have a poor outcome from CABG and require repeat surgery, which is nearly twice as expensive as the first operation and has a higher failure rate. Underwood and Bailey take the view that operating on CHD patients who persist in smoking 'deprives' patients who have never smoked or who quit smoking from access to treatment from which they have a higher chance of benefiting. These authors conclude that doctors have no obligation to subject smokers to a high-cost low-success procedure.

● What dilemmas are raised by Shiu?

■ He points to the doctors' ethical obligation to treat sick people on the basis of need with the best available treatment; he notes that if the same logic were to be applied to other conditions, then drunken victims of traffic accidents could be denied treatment unless they promised to give up alcohol, and so could people who attempt suicide. Denying CABG to smokers leads to the 'slippery slope' where doctors make value-judgements about deserving and undeserving cases.

8.4.4   Balancing prevention and treatment of CHD

The central dilemma raised at the start of this chapter is how to achieve the right balance between prevention, treatment and cure. In the case of CHD, there are no cures – only treatments. A pragmatic argument for adopting preventive strategies is that they may be more cost-effective than treating (or attempting unsuccessfully to treat) people who are already ill. If successful, then disease-prevention strategies would reduce the dependency associated with illness and hence produce other benefits to society as a whole, beyond the reduction in the cost of health and social services.

However, the question still remains of whether or not the total cost of 'case finding' and prevention is economically balanced against the benefit it provides (Box 8.1, principle 10). This question is particularly difficult when the total costs per person over a lifetime may *increase* because a consequence of preventing one disease is that individuals survive to develop other, costlier, illnesses.

Another possible dilemma arises from the recognition that most preventive services can only be offered, not enforced (Box 8.1, principle 6). Thus they may not reduce the *overall* incidence of disease in the population, but instead simply (and possibly expensively) be taken up only by the 'worried well' (a point made first in Chapter 2).

Getting the right balance between prevention and treatment depends on the relative effectiveness of the different strategies available, and that in turn requires accurate evaluation of their efficacy. We have already discussed various potential sources of bias in trials of secondary prevention strategies, such as the use of cholesterol-lowering drugs, and in the distribution of treatments such as CABG.

● What additional constraint limits the use of randomised controlled trials (RCTs) to evaluate *primary* prevention strategies? (If you are unsure, look back at the relevant section of Chapter 6.)

■ RCTs of interventions aimed at *preventing* disease take longer and need to have more people enlisted than do RCTs of medical treatments for *existing* disease. This is because to assess the effectiveness of any primary preventive strategy, rates have to be compared at which initially healthy people *become* ill or die in the intervention and control groups. Because not everyone *will* become ill, a much larger population sample is required to make a valid comparison, and they must be followed up for longer than when a medical treatment is subjected to an RCT in an already-ill population.

For example, for an RCT of a preventive intervention to have a reasonable chance of detecting a 10 per cent reduction in mortality that could be attributed to it, the trial might well require *30 000* people, each of them followed for *ten* years. A 10 per cent reduction in mortality for a *therapeutic* intervention might be as reliably detected with *3 000* patients followed for *two* years, because the outcome to be compared will usually be both more common and immediate. In the preventive comparison an 'outcome' event rate (such as death) of five per *thousand* per year would be considered high, whereas in the treatment comparison an event rate of five per *hundred* per year would be low.

However, many disease-prevention strategies, such as health education, cannot be assessed by RCTs at all, especially where they are non-medical in nature. And because prevention strategies are largely matters of public policy involving intersectoral collaboration between different local agencies and branches of central government, often requiring large amounts of public money, the evidence required to justify them must be especially accurate and compelling. By comparison, the standards of evidence required to justify new medical interventions are simpler to obtain and may be less rigorous, except in the evaluation of new drugs.

Policy decisions concerning the implementation of any preventive programme *should* depend on the careful assessment of costs and benefits, including opportunity costs. But because accurate evaluation is often difficult, even in huge studies such as the MONICA Project, decisions can still be made on political and ideological grounds, or on the basis of historical precedent and tradition (i.e. 'eminence-based' rather than 'evidence-based' medicine, as discussed in Chapter 6).

There are other reasons why the health-care sector is biased towards curative rather than preventive approaches to disease.[9]

● Can you suggest what these might be?

■ Illness is often frightening and painful to patients and carers alike, so every possible effort is usually made to alleviate individual suffering. Failure to provide immediate medical help for lives at risk is considered unethical in most situations. It might also lead to public protest and accusations of malpractice, which could undermine the prestige of the medical profession. That prestige is itself indicative of the dominance of curative medicine in Western culture; preventive medicine has a much lower status.

[9] See *Medical Knowledge: Doubt and Certainty* (Open University Press, 2nd edn 1994; colour-enhanced 2nd edn 2001) for a discussion of the prestige of medicine in Western culture; the dominance of specialist hospital medicine over public health or community medicine also has a long history, which is discussed in *Caring for Health: History and Diversity* (Open University Press, 3rd edn 2001).

Finally, the reasons for the declining trends in CHD in most industrialised countries are uncertain. The MONICA Project concluded that perhaps two-thirds of the reduction in deaths from CHD was due to falling coronary event rates, and one third was due to better survival among people who suffer a heart attack (Tunstall-Pedoe *et al.*, 1999). The decline in 'coronary events' could only partly be explained by reductions in risk factors, which in turn might be due to better prevention strategies (Kuulasmaa *et al.*, 2000). But an alternative explanation is that 'better prevention' is a marker for a wealthier economy and healthier early-life factors; it could be these social changes, rather than any interventions, that are responsible for the improving trends.

This case study on CHD has raised more questions than it has answered, but it illustrates for one important disease condition just how difficult it is to achieve meaningful gains in the nation's health. Many of the dilemmas explored here could be extrapolated to the prevention of other causes of death and disability.

8.5   Preventing disease: whose responsibility?

In the final section of this chapter, we return to the questions 'Who is responsible for protecting the nation's health?' and 'Can interference with individual freedoms be justified in preventing disease?'

These questions flow from divergent assumptions about the origins of ill health that can readily be distinguished. One type of approach assumes that the *individual* is responsible for his or her own health: it follows that the prevention of disease is consequent on individual behaviour *voluntarily* chosen, but stimulated and encouraged by relevant health education. In this version, people are left essentially free to choose their *lifestyle* and hence their level of health.

At the opposite extreme, the agencies of the *state* are held to be responsible for the nation's health: they can enforce healthier choices upon the population by *statutory* means (such as legislation enforcing the wearing of seat-belts, or banning smoking in public buildings), and sustain a health-promoting social, physical and economic *environment* through a network of public-health, fiscal and other policies. Somewhere between the two is an approach that incorporates elements of both individual and state action.

In practice, preventive measures directed at the individual and at the environment have the potential to complement one another: a ban on atmospheric pollutants, for example, not only compels individuals to change their behaviour, but also provides a healthier environment for everyone.

But as we noted in the introduction, many health-protection measures run the risk of crossing the boundary between acceptable and unacceptable infringement of people's liberty. And health education aimed at changing individual behaviour is open to criticism. If health is shaped by many different factors that fall outside the control of individuals, attempts to change individual behaviour will be undermined. The social climate in which individuals make health choices can also be influenced by powerful commercial interests, which (for example) promote products such as tobacco and alcohol as socially desirable even though they are detrimental to health.

Moves towards a 'community development' model of disease prevention, in which change is achieved through community action, appear to have a greater chance of success. However, given the criticisms of the concept of community that were rehearsed in Chapter 4, such an approach runs the danger of improving the health

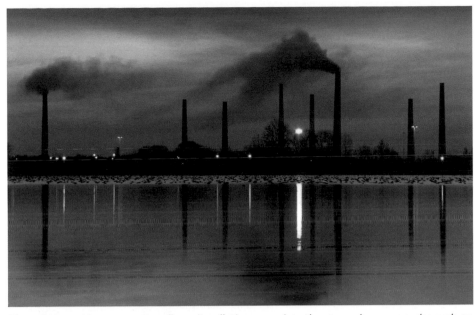

These factory chimneys continually emit polluting gases into the atmosphere; examples such as this call into question the extent to which individuals can be considered as able to take responsibility for their own health. (Photo: Mike Dodd)

of the more privileged members of society at the expense of those who are socially disadvantaged. And as you saw earlier, these are precisely the people who are most at risk from almost all manifestations of disease and disability.

Some public-health activists point to the clear association between poverty and ill health, and argue that only income redistribution and major legislative measures to alleviate social deprivation and improve environmental conditions will significantly improve the nation's health. It is to the dilemmas raised by anti-poverty strategies that we turn in the final chapter of this book.

OBJECTIVES FOR CHAPTER 8

When you have studied this chapter, you should be able to:

8.1 Define and use, or recognise definitions and applications of, each of the terms printed in **bold** in the text.

8.2 Discuss the principles involved in disease-prevention strategies at the primary, secondary and tertiary levels.

8.3 Illustrate the dilemmas inherent in disease-prevention strategies based on health-education campaigns, health-protection legislation, population screening and screening for high-risk individuals.

8.4 Summarise the classical risk factors associated with CHD, and explain why it is difficult to evaluate the evidence on potential causes and on the effectiveness of prevention programmes and treatments.

8.5 Discuss the possible contributions of socioeconomic and psychosocial factors to CHD rates, and comment on the implications for disease-prevention programmes.

QUESTIONS FOR CHAPTER 8

1   *(Objective 8.2)*

    Identify which of the following strategies is operating at the primary, secondary or tertiary levels of disease prevention and in each case explain your reasoning:

    • hip-replacement surgery for advanced arthritis in the hip joint;

    • legislation to reduce emission of smoke particles from industrial chimneys;

    • warnings on news bulletins about poor air quality;

    • 'childproof' caps on medicine bottles dispensed by pharmacies;

    • advice to limit salt intake as a means of reducing high blood pressure.

2   *(Objectives 8.3 and 8.4)*

    'A population screening programme to detect and treat individuals with raised cholesterol levels is likely to prove costly and ineffective in reducing death rates from CHD.'

    Discuss this statement in relation to national targets for reducing deaths from CHD in the UK. What ethical dilemmas does it raise?

3   *(Objective 8.4)*

    What are the main problems in determining the relative contributions of the classical risk factors to CHD rates in a country, and how do these problems make it more difficult to design effective CHD prevention and treatment programmes?

4   *(Objective 8.5)*

    What is the evidence that factors other than the classical risk factors for CHD need to be taken into account when designing CHD prevention programmes?

CHAPTER 9

Poverty, inequality, social exclusion and health

Study note for Open University students

Before reading this chapter, you should look back at Chapters 9 and 10 in *World Health and Disease* (Open University Press, 3rd edn 2001) to remind yourself of the nature of, and possible explanations for, inequalities in health in contemporary Britain. The video 'Status and wealth: the ultimate panacea?' and the audiotape 'Smoking: a global health problem', which were associated with that book, are also relevant to the present chapter, and you could usefully revise them now. In Section 9.6, you will be referred to an article entitled 'The psychosocial causes of illness', by Richard Wilkinson, which is optional reading and can be found in *Health and Disease: A Reader* (Open University Press, 3rd edn 2001). In Section 9.7, the conclusion of this chapter refers to another article in the Reader by D. R. Gwatkin, which is set reading for the course; it turns your attention from the UK focus of this book to the global context of 'Health inequalities and the health of the poor: What do we know? What can we do?'.

This chapter was jointly written by Mick Carpenter, Reader in Social Policy at the University of Warwick, and Alan Dolan, Lecturer in the School of Health and Social Studies at the University of Warwick.

9.1 Introduction

In Chapter 8, the complexity of coronary heart disease (CHD) illustrated how difficult it is for explanations of disease and disability to take account of all the potential contributing factors and the interactions between them. This book has demonstrated that strategies for alleviating or preventing complex health problems often produce dilemmas, and in this chapter we consider those that arise from strategies to reduce health inequalities. We move away from the confines of the health service to examine the recognition that poverty, inequality and social exclusion are powerful determinants of health, illness and disability in modern populations. This approach recognises that *health care* is very limited in the extent to which it can contribute to health improvement, or eliminate the social gradient in health.

Strategic responses aimed at reducing health inequalities will depend upon how deprivation is measured and also how the relationship between deprivation and health is understood. Dilemmas result from difficulties in agreeing on what to measure and how to intervene, which have already been introduced in the previous chapter in relation to reducing the rates of CHD.

The founding principles of the NHS enshrine the health-care and social-care systems as 'universal benefits' available equally to all, but this approach is open to the criticism that it is insufficiently focused on those in most need. However, replacing this system with one that is means-tested creates other dilemmas, not least because it threatens the principle of *equity* – that the benefit should be universal, regardless of means.

Since 1945, in the UK, there have been three contrasting and influential approaches to poverty reduction.

The first of these has been termed a *strategy of equality*, which sought from the 1940s to the 1970s to tackle poverty by redistributing income via the benefit system and providing universal services to all. The second, a *market approach to poverty*, emerged in the late 1970s and was motivated by anxiety about the negative effects of welfare spending and taxation on economic prosperity. It distinguished widening economic inequality from poverty, with the latter presumed to have been all but eliminated by improvements in living standards.

Finally, with the election of a Labour government in 1997, a *strategy of social inclusion* emerged, which acknowledged that poverty had increased in step with widening economic inequality. This new approach distanced itself from both the 'strategy of equality' and the 'market approach', and favoured targeted measures to enhance poor people's access to jobs through skills training and education.

This chapter begins with a brief review of the evidence for inequalities in health in the UK and their possible explanations. It then moves on to consider the current debates surrounding the meaning, scale and causes of poverty and economic inequality and the evidence that suggests that the number of people living in poverty has increased significantly since the 1980s. Next we discuss the extent to which the increase in poverty may be linked to the strategic policies designed to address the problem from the late 1970s to the 1990s (as outlined above), before turning to consider how far anti-poverty policy shifted in a new direction after the election of a Labour government in 1997. Finally, we examine the extent to which the strategy of social inclusion is likely to reduce poverty, social inequality and inequalities in health and illness. We ask how effective these strategies will be in improving the health of individuals and what will be their impact on the general health of the UK population.

Overarching all of this analysis is the tension between the creation and the redistribution of wealth, which has been a major feature of political debates both inside and outside the health system since long before the founding of the NHS.

9.2   Social inequalities in health

Patterns of health and disease among people are not randomly distributed. There are distinct and persistent inequalities in the distribution of premature death, illness and disability in the UK, which have continued despite a general increase in prosperity and overall reductions in mortality. Inequalities in health exist whether socio-economic position is defined by the Registrar-General's definition of social class based on occupation, or on income, education, housing tenure or locality.

There is substantial evidence to show that those who live in more disadvantaged circumstances suffer more illness and have shorter lives than other people. For instance, Shaw and colleagues (1999) have compared the areas with the 'best health' and 'worst health' in the UK and found that people living in the 'worst health' areas, who also tend to be the poorest, were 2.6 times more likely to die before the age of 65 than those living in the 'best health' areas.

However, it is important to recognise that a **social gradient in health** exists, in which people's social and material circumstances reflect their health status at each point on the gradient. Although the 'health gap' between those at the top and those at the bottom of the scale has been given most publicity, people in intermediate circumstances also have intermediate health indicators.

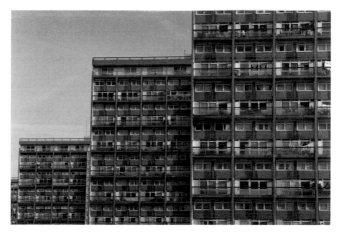

It is likely that the health of people living in these high-rise blocks of flats will be worse than the health of people who live in leafy suburbs. There is also evidence to show the existence of distinct inequalities between adjacent streets. (Photo: John Harris/Report Digital)

● What does this tell us about the link between people's circumstances and their health?

■ It demonstrates that even when people have a moderate level of income and other social and material factors, they suffer some health disadvantage compared with people in better circumstances. The obvious conclusion is that 'inequalities in health' affect the *majority* of the population, not just those who live in poverty.

Recent evidence from the Office for National Statistics also shows that inequalities in health have worsened in recent years:

> Life expectancy has increased for all social classes since 1972 but this disguises increasing inequality. For men the difference in life expectancy at birth between social classes I (professional occupations) and V (unskilled manual occupations) has risen from 5.5 years in 1972–76 to 9.5 years by 1996. The difference for women has risen from 5.3 years to 6.4 years. (Hattersley, 1999, p. 24)

● Suggest some explanations for these inequalities in health.[1]

■ The four most prominent explanations are that health inequalities are the result of:

an *artefact* of the statistics themselves;

social selection, whereby less healthy individuals move down the social hierarchy, and more healthy individuals move up;

cultural–behavioural effects of lifestyle choices of individuals and groups;

material inequalities in the circumstances of different social groups.

The weight of evidence now firmly supports the view that, although biological characteristics and individual lifestyles have a role to play, people's material circumstances are the *major* determinants of inequalities in health and illness. In Chapter 8, evidence for inequalities in the distribution of CHD was reported from the Whitehall Studies of all grades of staff, from managers to porters, employed in the civil service. The combined findings of these continuing studies reveal that for *all* major causes of death, those in lower employment grades had higher mortality rates than those in higher grades (van Rossum *et al.*, 2000).

However, even when all of the material factors are controlled for, there is a substantial residual disadvantage in being 'poor', which cannot be accounted for by material deprivation. Furthermore, even when all the known risk factors for specific diseases were excluded (e.g. smoking, obesity, lack of exercise), a significant difference in health experience between highest and lowest employment grades remained. The underlying causes of this residual disadvantage are the subject of intensive research, which points to the health-damaging effects of having low control over the circumstances of one's life, including in the workplace for those with low-paid jobs, leading to low self-esteem and a sense of being unvalued by the surrounding society.

Measures to combat inequalities in health faced by disadvantaged groups and communities figure prominently in the 1999 government White Paper, *Saving Lives: Our Healthier Nation* (in Scotland, *Scottish Health: Working together for a healthier Scotland*; in Northern Ireland, *Well into 2000*; and in Wales, *Better health, better Wales*). This was the first government policy document not only to acknowledge explicitly the links between poverty and health, but also to suggest that only by tackling poverty and social issues associated with poverty – most significantly unemployment – can improvements in the health of all be made. What is clear is that the relationship between poverty, inequality and social exclusion is complex, and consequently any political solution will not be straightforward.

9.3   Defining and measuring poverty

Debates about the nature and causes of poverty have continued ever since Seebohm Rowntree conducted his first survey of town life in 1901. This is more than an issue of semantics, as MacPherson and Silburn observe:

> … the seemingly academic questions of poverty — definition and measurement — have profound consequences for policy and practice, and thus for those now condemned to poverty and its consequences. (MacPherson and Silburn, 1998, p.117)

[1] The evidence for the four explanations referred to in the answer to this question were discussed in *World Health and Disease* (Open University Press, 3rd edn 2001), Chapter 10. Explanations 3 and 4 have been exemplified many times in books in the 'Health and Disease' series, including in Chapter 8 of the present book.

The adoption of a narrow focus on poverty, as something which is 'absolute', or a more inclusive acceptance that poverty is 'relative', will affect the extent to which we believe 'the poor' should have either restricted or wider claims on society, and the *threshold of decency* that society is prepared to tolerate. It raises the dilemma of which measure of poverty we should use in order to address inequalities in health. How these measures are devised and applied is therefore a crucial first step in achieving this goal.

9.3.1 Poverty as absolute or relative?

The concept of **absolute poverty** is based upon the notion of bare subsistence — the minimum standards of food, shelter and clothing necessary to sustain life — and occurs when people fall below this minimum. For example, Sir Keith Joseph, a former Conservative Secretary of State for Social Services, argued that:

> A family is poor if it cannot afford to eat. A person who enjoys a standard of living equal to that of a medieval baron cannot be described as poor for the sole reason that he has chanced to be born into a society where the great majority can live like medieval kings. By any absolute standards, there is very little poverty. (Joseph and Sumption, 1979, p. 27)

This restrictive approach is challenged by those who suggest that poverty can be defined only relatively (**relative poverty**), that is in relation to particular social contexts, because living standards and needs change over time. They argue that people need resources not just to subsist but also to participate in the life of the community. Peter Townsend (one of the authors of the Black Report on health inequalities, DHSS, London, 1980) has long sought to elaborate such an approach and define it systematically in terms of **deprivation**:

> Individuals, families and groups in the population can be said to be in poverty when they lack the resources to obtain the types of diet, participate in the activities and have the living conditions and amenities which are customary ... in the societies to which they belong. (Townsend, 1979, p.131)

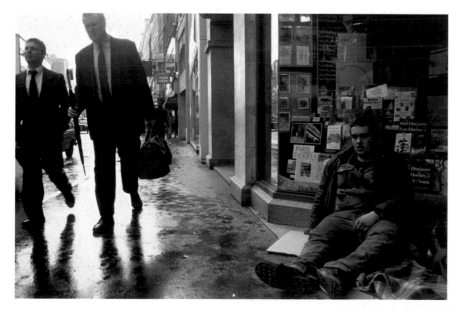

Being homeless and sleeping on the streets became an increasingly common sight in Britain in the 1980s and 1990s. Strategies to remove people from the streets were also strategies to remove the sight of 'absolute' poverty. (Photo: Gideon Mendel/ Network)

Within this definition, poverty is thus a lack of *material* resources that prevents people not just from enjoying a certain level of consumption, but also from participating as 'citizens' in the life of the community.

The development of the concept of relative poverty played a crucial role in the 1960s in establishing a new agenda for debates about poverty, casting doubt on the belief that the welfare state had eliminated it. For example, although state benefits may be sufficient for bare subsistence (though there is some argument about this), they have not maintained parity with average earnings. This became increasingly important in the 1980s and 1990s, when greater numbers of people were dependent on benefits as a sole source of income.

● Identify a dilemma in adopting either an absolute or a relative approach to the definition of poverty.

■ As far as absolute poverty is concerned, how do we decide what people could do without, for example is a daily newspaper or a television set a 'necessity'? With regard to relative poverty, how far should we go in viewing access to a customary standard of living as a 'right'?

Although an absolute approach may at first sight appear the more objective, both approaches necessarily involve value judgements about social entitlements. In any case, in practice so-called absolute approaches cannot avoid including items that are socially necessary rather than required for bare subsistence. Thus, Rowntree's surveys between 1901 to 1951, which established subsistence standards for state benefits, tended towards stringency by particular emphasis on food items and housing costs, but Rowntree accepted that buying a newspaper was socially necessary. However, he did not approve of poor people spending money on gambling or beer. These were of course essentially social and moral judgements, as was his distinction between **primary poverty** – where by his strict standards people were deemed to be genuinely poor – and **secondary poverty**, where people were said to have sufficient but did not spend their money wisely.

9.3.2 A social consensus on poverty

If it is accepted that poverty can be defined only in relation to a changing way of life within a society (in this case the UK), it may be possible to reach a measure of public agreement about how poverty should be defined. This was the approach first used in a population survey in 1983 by Joanna Mack and Stewart Lansley, in which they sought to investigate the extent of a subjective social consensus around relative poverty (Mack and Lansley, 1985). Subsequently this survey was updated for the television series 'Breadline Britain 1990s' (Frayman, 1991). A large representative sample of people across the UK were asked what items they regarded as necessities or luxuries, and the results revealed a surprising level of agreement. There was also a tendency for particular items, such as telephones and fridges, to shift increasingly from luxury to necessity status between the two surveys. By the 1990s, at least two-thirds of those asked regarded the items in Box 9.1 as necessities.

> **Box 9.1   Items regarded as necessities by at least two-thirds of adults surveyed for the TV series 'Breadline Britain 1990s'**
>
> - Self-contained damp-free accommodation with an indoor toilet and bath
> - A weekly roast joint for the family and three daily meals for each child
> - Two pairs of all-weather shoes and a warm waterproof coat
> - Sufficient money for public transport
> - Adequate bedrooms and beds
> - Heating and carpeting
> - A refrigerator and a washing machine
> - Enough money for special occasions like Christmas
> - Toys for the children.
>
> Source: Frayman, H. (1991) *Breadline Britain 1990s*, Domino Films/London Weekend Television, p. 4.

Mack and Lansley defined poverty as a situation where people had to live without three or more of the items that society as a whole regarded as necessities. Using this index as a framework for measuring poverty among their sample, they found that around 20 per cent of households, containing 11 million people — including 3 million children — were in poverty in 1991. This represented an increase of almost 50 per cent compared with 1983, when they had found 14 per cent of households, approximately 7.5 million people, living in poverty.

This approach is innovative in that it removes definitions from the experts in order to 'let the people decide' — but *only* on the items that the researchers have selected for the survey. The broader set of necessities advocated by Mack and Lansley also implicitly hangs on to Rowntree's distinction between *primary* and *secondary* poverty, though it is more generous about what items are to be included. An alternative approach, beginning to gain ground in a number of countries, is to develop research instruments that ask people themselves to identify what they need to sustain a customary way of life.

● What is the advantage of this approach to defining relative poverty?

■ It is focused more directly on people's own perceived requirements of what they need to avoid being 'poor', and thus can be adapted to various societies with very different living standards and cultures.

9.3.3 The state benefit 'safety net'

Another method of defining poverty takes account of the provision of state benefits to people on low, or no income. A **relative poverty line** can be drawn at the point at which benefit support from the state is paid. Inevitably there is disagreement about whether the line is drawn in the right place, and the arguments centre on what people on benefits should be able to afford for a 'decent' minimum standard of living. Thus, state benefit is often described as a *safety net* put in place to stop people from 'falling' out of mainstream society and into the underclass of those in poverty.

According to the income support/benefit standard of entitlement, approximately 8 per cent of UK households or 4.75 million people in 1992 lived below this 'poverty line', which represented an increase of only 2 per cent on 1979 figures (Oppenheim and Harker, 1996).

● What is the main drawback of using the provision of state benefits as a measure of poverty?

■ Changes in government policy and fluctuations in the national economic climate can influence the level of income at which eligibility for benefits begins; whenever this notional poverty line is moved down (i.e. made less 'generous'), people are taken out of the technical definition of poverty because they are no longer eligible for state benefits, even though their material circumstances have not changed

Similarly, benefit levels were pegged to price rises during a period when earnings rose more rapidly.

9.3.4 Trends in household income

It could be argued that a better marker for relative poverty is **households below average income** (HBAI). This measures the number of people living on incomes below half the national average, but it uses household income, adjusted for household size after allowing for housing costs. HBAI is a better reflection of living standard than average individual earnings, because it takes account of household composition. It has become the customary means of making comparisons among partners in the European Union.

Trends in HBAI over time in the UK are represented in Figure 9.1, while Table 9.1 shows the political complexion of UK governments since 1945.

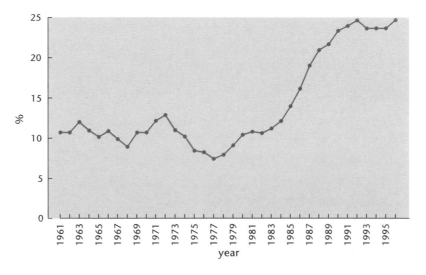

Figure 9.1 *Percentage of the UK population living in households whose total income was below half average income (after housing costs) (1961–96) (Source: Gordon, D., 2000, Inequalities in Income, Wealth and Standard of Living in Britain, in Pantazis, C. and Gordon, D. (eds)* Tackling Inequalities: Where Are We Now and What Can Be Done?, *Policy Press, Bristol, Figure 2.2, p. 32)*

HBAI for 1996 (the final year covered in Figure 9.1) shows that 25 per cent of the UK population was living in households on incomes below half the national average. Table 9.1 lists the changes in political parties forming UK governments since 1945.

Table 9.1 UK governments since 1945 by political party.

1945–51	Labour
1951–64	Conservative
1964–70	Labour
1970–74	Conservative
1974–79	Labour
1979–97	Conservative
1997–	Labour

● On the basis of Figure 9.1 and Table 9.1, what are the main trends in relative poverty since the 1960s, and how do they map against the political changes listed?

■ Relative poverty rose in the early 1960s when a Conservative government was in office. Though it fell initially when Labour came into power in 1964, it had risen again to around its former level by the time that Labour left office in 1970. It continued rising in the first years of Conservative rule, but had started to fall before Labour came into office in 1974, and continued to fall for most of the 1970s. The most striking feature is the steep increase in relative poverty since the late 1970s, in the long period of Conservative government that ended in 1997. It rose from a low point of around 7 per cent in 1978 to reach 25 per cent in 1996, the year before Labour was re-elected.

By 1996, more than 12.2 million people in the UK, nearly 4 million of them children, were living in relative poverty (Eurostat, 1997).

● What causal explanation might be suggested for the relationship shown between Figure 9.1 and Table 9.1?

■ One possible explanation is that the welfare and employment policies of different governments could affect the level of poverty directly (an issue we will return to later in this chapter).

However, it is an elementary rule of statistics to be cautious about imputing causes between two correlated variables. In the situation represented by Figure 9.1 and Table 9.1, you should not automatically assume that it is the action of governments alone that lead the levels of relative poverty to rise or fall.

This raises the problem of how anti-poverty strategies can be effective when they are changed in the short term by political parties, but when their efficacy needs to be assessed over the longer term. Short-term strategies and long-term effects make it even more difficult to disaggregate the multiple interacting causes of poverty and to devise effective interventions to reduce inequalities in health.

A focus on relative poverty raises wider dilemmas of social justice; not just whether poor people have enough to live on, but also the essential 'fairness' of the social order. Is it fair that some people are living so far below the poverty line, however that is drawn? Is it the moral duty of society to redistribute wealth and to equalise people's chances, or are individuals responsible for their own health and welfare?

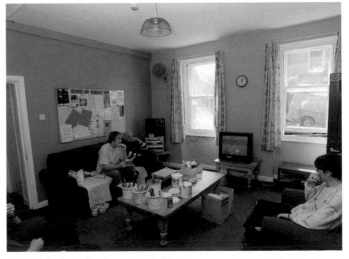

Part of the strategy to reduce poverty has been to provide homeless people with physical shelter as a basic material need. This hostel in Sheffield is typical of many that provide shelter for younger people. (Photo: Mike Levers)

In summary, there is no single universally accepted way of measuring poverty; ethical and political judgements necessarily intervene in decisions about where and how to draw the poverty line. Nevertheless, the general adoption of an absolute subsistence or a relative approach has important practical implications, not least in affecting the numbers deemed to be poor, and thus the extent to which poverty is judged to be an urgent issue of public concern.

9.3.5 Who are 'the poor'?

By all accounts, since the 1980s, the UK has become an increasingly unequal society. However, the data presented so far do not tell the whole story. In order to reduce inequalities in health we need to know who is most at risk of poverty, why they are vulnerable, and whether the causes have changed over time.

Whereas some people move in and out of poverty, others experience it over a prolonged period. It is also the case, as Rowntree recognised, that more people experience poverty than are poor at any one time. He described a 'cycle of poverty' associated with working class life, which led people to move below the poverty line at particularly vulnerable stages in the life course — as a child, as an adult with family responsibilities for children, and when earning capacity disappeared after retirement age.

We can start to explore these issues by examining Table 9.2.

Table 9.2   The risk of poverty: by family and economic status 1994–95.

UK population group	Percentage of each category of households with incomes below HBAI/%
By family status:	
pensioner, couple	24
pensioner, single	32
couple with children	22
couple without children	10
single with children	60
single without children	22
By economic status:	
self-employed	22
single or couple, all in full-time work	2
one in full-time work, one in part-time work	3
one in full-time work, one not working	17
one or more in part-time work	33
head or spouse aged 60 or over	29
head or spouse unemployed	74
other	61

Source: George, V. and Wilding, P. (1999) *British Society and Social Welfare*, Macmillan, London, Table 5.7, p. 140.

Table 9.2 distinguishes between the composition of the poor by family status and by economic status, and presents the risk of poverty as measured by HBAI. It is the proportion of each category at risk of poverty (as defined by HBAI) that is important.

● From the data in Table 9.2, which categories of people are most 'at risk' of poverty? (For the purposes of this discussion, you can discount the small number of people whose economic status could not be determined and is given as 'other'.)

■ 74 per cent of households in which the 'head' of household is unemployed are living on incomes below half the average; a majority of single-parent families (60 per cent) are also 'poor' by HBAI definition.

Although these two categories stand out, it is notable that 'pensioners', part-time workers and also self-employed people have a higher risk of experiencing below-average household income than others. Note that poverty and inequality exist not only between groups, but also within them. Relatively few households are at risk of poverty where there are no children and/or one or more adult is in full-time work and the other is also employed.

9.3.6 Poverty, wealth and life chances

At the beginning of this chapter we referred to the social gradient in health and the fact that material circumstances are strongly associated with health status at all points from top to bottom of the social scale, however this is measured.

Against this background, **wealth**, defined as a combination of income and assets, is also relevant to understanding issues of inequality in health. Thus, although income is a useful measure of a person's current economic situation, their access to wealth beyond earnings is also relevant. For many people the most important asset they own is their house, but this is often mortgaged. They might also have an occupational pension, but this cannot be immediately accessed. A minority of people, however, own outright substantial amounts of property and land, and have wealth invested in abstract forms of capital, such as share ownership, which can be sold off at any time. Like income, the ownership of wealth is therefore unequally distributed.

The widening gap between rich and poor is also evident in the distribution of wealth, although accurate data on the latter are not always easy to obtain. Hills (1998) found that from the 1940s up to 1980, inequality in wealth distribution saw a significant narrowing and income inequality also reduced in this period; but since the 1980s income inequality has widened while the distribution of wealth appears to have changed little. However, this is not the whole picture: if *housing* is excluded from the definition of wealth, then inequalities in wealth have become significantly wider since the 1980s. On this basis, David Gordon (2000, pp. 39–40) has calculated that in 1976, the top 10 per cent of the UK population owned 57 per cent of the national wealth; by 1994 they owned 65 per cent of the nation's wealth. The poorest 10 per cent of people owned approximately 2 per cent of the nation's income and even less of the nation's wealth.

● There are also 'non-cash' resources that can be included in definitions of wealth. Can you suggest some of them?

■ People who are 'better off' have enhanced access to amenities like pleasant, less polluted streets and parks, by virtue of where they live; they can also reach out-of-town shops and supermarkets accessible only by car. They may also gain access to benefits in kind for themselves and their kin through occupational welfare, such as pension schemes, private health care, social clubs and other facilities.

If you couple these benefits with the greater opportunities, 'life chances' and social esteem generally experienced by people in comfortable material circumstances, and add the relative autonomy allowed to people in most well-paid jobs, it becomes easier to understand how wealth and health could be associated.

In theory, the tax and benefits system serves to redistribute wealth and reduce the 'wealth gap'. Similarly, the taxation system operates in an egalitarian fashion in relation to funding universal health and social services and education, in that everyone who is employed makes a regular contribution that is deducted at source. A proportion of the National Insurance charge goes directly to fund the NHS.

However, there is evidence that redistribution of wealth by taxation has regressed in Britain since the 1980s. According to estimates from the Low Pay Unit (1999), between 1983 and 1995 the taxes on household income fell from 41 to 36 per cent for the richest fifth, and rose from 27 to 39 per cent for the poorest fifth. Rather than redistributing wealth according to a system of need, it would appear that those who are less well off were further disadvantaged by taxation in this period. Despite this, social security plays a significant role in cushioning temporary poverty as well as helping the 'long-term poor', but the need to eradicate the causes of poverty remains an important long-term goal in any public health programme.

This housing estate is one that has good access to schools, shops and transport. The area is also one of high employment. Capital wealth is not the only benefit enjoyed by the people who live here. (Photo: Joy Wilson)

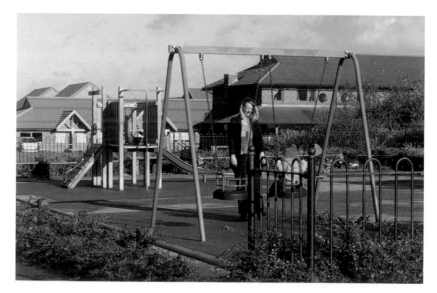

9.4   The causes of poverty and inequality

Figure 9.1 showed the rapid rise in relative poverty from the later 1970s onwards. In 1998, the Report of the Joseph Rowntree Foundation Inquiry *Income and Wealth* (Hills, 1998), highlighted the following factors underlying this trend:

• The gap between low and high incomes widened between 1979 and 1994–95.

Thus, in terms of *real* (i.e. not just relative) incomes after housing costs, the poorest 10 per cent of households experienced a cut of 8 per cent, while average household incomes increased by 43 per cent, and the top 10 per cent of households increased their incomes by 68 per cent. In other words, those households that comprise the middle group increased their incomes, but the 'poorest' got relatively 'poorer' and the 'rich' got relatively 'richer', so the gap between the top and bottom widened.

- Unemployment — and numbers receiving benefits — rose rapidly in this period.

Importantly, the number of households without anyone in work rose faster than unemployment as a whole. This was partly due to the growth in the number of single parents. In addition, because at the time of writing in 2001 the social security system treats 'two adult' households as a single unit and withdraws benefit if one of them works more than a few hours a week, there is a growing polarisation between 'no-earner' and 'two-earner' households.

- Arrangements for uprating benefit levels widened the gap between benefit claimants and wage earners.

Income support became linked to the Retail Price Index, which rose more slowly than earnings, and hence those reliant on benefits automatically fell behind those on earnings.

9.4.1 Structural divisions in society

The rapid rise of poverty in the UK since the 1980s has meant that those people who were already disadvantaged by social divisions, such as class, gender and ethnicity, have been more likely to remain at a comparatively 'poorer' position within these groups. The evidence of cumulative disadvantage in health terms from being in such a position is now compelling.

It is more than likely that the majority of those who move in and out of poverty are, in terms of occupation, people from social classes IV and V — particularly those who are unskilled and unqualified on the margins of the labour market — whether in work or not. And it must not be forgotten that people from black and Asian ethnic groups are over-represented in these social class categories, and fare badly in health terms in comparison with the majority white population (a point we return to below). The risks of poverty and illness remain sharply class-related in British society.

9.4.2 Women and poverty

Women are more at risk of being in poverty than are men, partly because single-parent households are most often headed by women and these are among the poorest families (as Table 9.2 showed). However, the full extent of women's poverty has generally remained hidden, particularly in studies based on household income.

- ● Why might such studies disguise women's poverty?

- ■ They ignore the fact that poverty can occur *within* families where the total income brings the household above the poverty line. Women are particularly vulnerable to this disadvantage.

Within households, individuals may remain relatively poor through inequitable distribution of income and other resources (Millar and Glendinning, 1992). Table 9.3 (*overleaf*) makes a comparison between the causes of poverty in both sexes and among women. It also compares the results of the Rowntree poverty study carried out in York in 1899, with data for Britain in 1987 collected by the Department of Social Security (DSS). The data are thought to be sufficiently representative for these comparisons to be valid.

Table 9.3 Comparison of causes of poverty among both sexes and among women, York 1899 and Britain 1987. [a]

	Among both sexes		Among women	
	1899 (York poverty study data)/%	1987 (DSS data)/%	1899 (York poverty study data)/%	1987 (DSS data)/%
Old age, sickness and disability	12	32	22	49
One-parent family	9	15	18	14
Unemployment	5	31	6	23
Large family[b]	22	14	14	6
Low wages	52	8	40	8
Totals	100	100	100	100

[a] The major cause of poverty was determined by the researchers. Note that the categories of 'old age', 'sickness' and 'disability' are not mutually exclusive.

[b] 1899 = families with five or more children; 1987 = three or more children.

Source: Lewis, J. and Piachaud, D. (1992) Women and Poverty in the Twentieth Century, in Glendinning, C. and Millar, J. (eds) *Women and Poverty in Britain in the 1990s*, Harvester Wheatsheaf, Hemel Hempstead, Table 3.5, p. 42.

● Which causes of poverty among women have changed in importance between 1899 and 1987, according to Table 9.3?

■ Old age, sickness and disability had become a far more prevalent cause of female poverty by 1987, and so had unemployment; conversely, low wages had diminished sharply in importance, and there were smaller declines in the other causes between the two dates.

Unemployment, relatively low at the turn of the century, increased in the 1930s but fell from the 1940s, only to rise in prominence again in the 1980s. Although it is a more significant cause of poverty among men, it remains prominent as a cause among women. Low pay was a prime cause of poverty in 1899 for both sexes but appears to have fallen among both men and women. Family relationships have remained important, but in different ways. For example, as the twentieth century progressed, women were increasingly able to regulate their fertility to the extent that family size is a less significant influence on poverty. Conversely, the rates of divorce and single parenthood have increased.

However, the question remains: why should old age, sickness and disability be associated particularly with poverty among women? To provide a full explanation, we need to look in a detailed way at women's structural position in society.

The number of full-time low-paid workers in Britain rose from 28.3 to 37 per cent of the total workforce between 1979 and 1994, using the **Council of Europe's decency threshold** of 68 per cent of average earnings to define 'low paid'. Part-time work, which is particularly associated with women's work and usually paid at a lower hourly rate than full-time work, increased significantly during this period. Furthermore, pay among full-time working women in the same period fell from 58 to 50 per cent of average earnings (Evans, 1998, pp. 266–7).

Relatively speaking, the pay of most men exceeds that of women by a substantial margin. Data for 1996–97 show that, typically, women's income peaks at an average of £200 a week in their early 20s, and then starts to decline to an average of around £100 a week from age 60 onwards. Men's income, however, tends to increase to an average of £400 a week between 45 and 50, before gradually declining thereafter (Office for National Statistics, 2000b, pp. 84–5).

● Why should this 'averaging' approach be treated with caution?

■ The problem is that it does not show the extent of diversity in income *within* each sex.

However, it demonstrates that the average lifetime earnings of women is far outstripped by that of men. The extent to which the relative disadvantage in terms of income and wealth experienced by women has consequences for their health is uncertain. What is not in dispute is that women on average live longer than men but experience (or at least report) greater morbidity, particularly from depression and other psychological disorders. This pattern of illness reflects the social gradient, with women lower down the poverty scale experiencing more ill health than women in better circumstances.[2]

9.4.3 Ethnicity and poverty

Table 9.4 shows that the risk of poverty is closely associated with ethnicity. For example, 47 per cent of white households where no members were in work were in poverty (according to the definition used in this study), but 75 per cent of unemployed Pakistani and Bangladeshi households were considered poor. In all households, the likelihood of black and other ethnic minority people experiencing poverty was significantly greater than for white people, and this is linked to other forms of disadvantage, such as low pay and unemployment.

What is also striking, however, is that these risks were much greater for people from Pakistani and Bangladeshi backgrounds, whether they were in or out of work. This has been confirmed by other research which shows that, while 23 per cent of 'white' families earn one-and-a-half times the average household income, 12 per cent of Caribbean and only 1.5 per cent of Pakistanis and Bangladeshis did so (Modood *et al.*, 1997).

Table 9.4 Percentage of households in Great Britain below 60 per cent average income by economic status and ethnic group, 1996–98. [a]

Type of household	White/%	Black[b]/%	Indian/%	Pakistani and Bangladeshi/%	All/%
All above pension age	24	–	–	–	24
Other households:					
no members in work	47	52	55	75	49
at least one member in work	9	–	20	56	10
All households	17	28	27	64	18

[a] Data from the Family Resources Survey, a continuous survey with a sample size of 341 502 households. (Source: Office for National Statistics, 2000, *Social Trends 30*, Table 5.20, p. 94)

[b] 'Black' refers to all ethnic minority groups other than Indian, Pakistani and Bangladeshi.

[2] A discussion of work and health in adult life, which refers to the effects on working women of the 'double day' (domestic chores and childcare, alongside employment outside the home), occurs in *Birth to Old Age: Health in Transition* (Open University Press, colour-enhanced 2nd edn 2001), Chapter 8.

In sum, the most important causes of poverty are related first to the current access of household members to paid work in the labour market, and secondly, the presence or absence of children in the household. These in turn are connected to social processes linked to divisions of class, gender, and ethnicity.

9.5 Strategies for tackling poverty

9.5.1 The social and economic climate

There is considerable debate about whether growing social divisions are spontaneously generated, or have been deliberately or unintentionally fostered by government policies. It is undoubtedly the case that welfare needs have increased and the ability of national welfare states to meet them has decreased. The kinds of social and economic development that may have had an influence include:

- Demographic shifts to low birth rate and increased life expectancy, leading to a growing number of older people, although the poverty gap among older people remains.

- Social changes, such as increased numbers of divorces and a rise in single parenthood, leading to greater numbers of women entering the workforce.

- Technological changes reducing the demand for low-skilled labour in manufacturing, creating a smaller 'core' of secure, better-paid manufacturing jobs.

- Employment shifts towards the service industry and multiplication of low-paid, often part-time and insecure jobs in services such as shops, restaurants and cleaning.

- Globalization of finance markets and multinational companies reducing the power of trade unions, and their ability to defend jobs.

These changes cannot be seen as entirely independent of political and cultural influences, as they have had different impacts in different countries. In particular, they are more associated with the growth of poverty and inequality in Britain and the USA than in continental Europe, indicating that policy choices have played a part.

In the rest of this section, we review the major trends in policy that have addressed the problem of poverty in the UK since the inception of the welfare state after World War II.

9.5.2 A strategy of equality

In Britain, in the decades following the Beveridge Index Report (1942), the response to poverty was what Richard Tawney, one of the twentieth-century architects of the welfare state, claimed to be a **strategy of equality**. The belief was that male, full employment would result in a universal social security system. What this meant in practice was that money collected in the form of taxes and contributions from those in paid employment would provide benefits to those categories of people — the unemployed, sick or retired — who are most at risk of poverty. It was primarily intended as a scheme for the protection of those outside the labour market, as the Beveridge approach assumed that waged employment would prevent poverty not just for the 'male breadwinner' but also 'his wife and children'. This would however be supplemented by benefits such as state pensions and adequate child allowances (Child Benefit), together with public expenditure in the fields of health, education and housing.

Economic prosperity and full male employment in the 1950s and 1960s sustained this approach. This prosperity faltered as *relative* poverty increased and critics showed that the welfare state was of most benefit to the middle class. Then the oil recessions of the 1970s heralded the end of the long post-war boom.[3]

9.5.3 Market approaches

In Chapter 1 you read about the role that ideologies play in structuring the system of health care. Support for a strategy that would redistribute resources more equitably has not endured in the UK, which is a society based on the principles of liberal democracy. In such a society 'individualism' is given a privileged status and the pursuit of collective ideals is often denigrated, particularly where this would require state intervention and central planning. An ideology based on individualism states that wealth is generated by individual efforts and abilities and that removing the incentive of potential wealth would result in a reduction in wealth generation. Supporters of this view argue that the long-term consequence would be a worsening of everyone's health and wealth.

This ideology is evident in a significant shift in economic policy by the Conservative governments of the 1980s and 1990s, which has become known as the **market approach**. The control of inflation took precedence over full employment as the economic strategy. However, inflation control was never intended as an instrument to affect poverty directly. The argument was that, unless inflation was curbed, more people would lose employment and become poor. A system of incentives to create wealth, such as incentives to work and to buy property, emerged. Social security was seen *not* as a means for preventing poverty, but as a drain on economic development and the economy. Conservative politicians of this period argued that the welfare state seduced recipients into a 'dependency culture', undermined people's willingness to work and maintain traditional family structures, and also explained the rise in divorce and single parenthood.

The very *existence* of poverty was disputed by some leading politicians in this period, claiming that the success of capitalism had put an end to poverty in the absolute sense of hunger and want. John Moore (1989), as Secretary of State for Social Security, in a keynote speech on social welfare, attacked the poverty lobby for continuing to promote the notion of relative poverty. He refuted the claim that large numbers of the population were living on the margins of poverty, and challenged the equation of poverty with inequality rather than with 'starving children and squalid slums'. He went on to say:

> We [the Conservative government] reject their claims about poverty in the UK, and we do so knowing that their motive is not compassion for the less well-off …. Their purpose in calling 'poverty' what is in reality simply inequality, is so they can call western capitalism a failure. (Moore, 1989, p.114)

From this vision, successive Conservative governments of the 1980s and early 1990s sought to 'roll back' the state, in an attempt both to cut welfare expenditure and to force people to take responsibility for themselves. Welfare policy shifted towards greater *selectivity* in targeting the 'genuinely' needy, most obviously by a succession of cutbacks in National Insurance benefits (which became the Job Seekers'

---

[3] The effects of the retrenchment in the UK health service which followed the 1970s oil crisis are described in *Caring for Health: History and Diversity* (Open University Press, 3rd edn 2001), Chapters 1 and 7.

Allowance) and increased reliance on means-tested benefits. The solution to poverty would come, it was argued, not from redistribution of resources towards the poor, but through a market approach associated with incentives to create wealth and a focus on the individual, leading to economic growth and general economic prosperity. The increased resources would gradually 'trickle down' to improve the living standards of those at the bottom. So while inequality would increase, the poor would benefit.

● Was this expectation fulfilled?

■ As you saw earlier, the incomes of the poorest 10 per cent of the population actually fell in real terms during this period.

9.5.4 Social inclusion

Debates about the need to include people who have been marginalised through material deprivation have been ongoing since the 1960s, and again became topical in the 1990s.

After winning the election of May 1997, the Labour government gave considerable priority to poverty and its effects on health. However, it was primarily the twin notions of **social exclusion** and **welfare to work** that distinguished the government's approach to groups such as the unemployed, single parents and disabled people. The idea that poverty leads to social exclusion was adopted initially from European Union social policy approaches, which extend the notion of relative poverty to embrace a wider concept of personal resources, and to identify the social processes that produce poverty and marginalise the poor:

> Exclusion processes are dynamic and multidimensional in nature. They are linked not only to unemployment and/or to low incomes, but also to housing conditions, levels of education and opportunities, health, discrimination, citizenship and integration into the local community. (European Social Policy White Paper (1994), cited in Oppenheim and Harker, 1996, p. 156)

This approach is broadly consistent with Townsend's definition of relative poverty, which includes income and other forms of deprivation and prevents people from participating in the customary social life of their community.

Considerable emphasis was placed on reform of the benefit system, in particular on welfare-to-work training programmes designed to ease the passage into employment, underpinned by the introduction of a 'competitive' minimum wage, the Working Families Tax Credit, and other incentives such as help with child-care costs and the expansion of pre-school nursery places. Paid work was seen as a way to reduce poverty and any associated sense of 'uselessness', and so the social inclusion strategy aimed to remove some of the barriers to work while reducing the acceptability of state dependence. The government made it clear that the state's role in preventing poverty and social exclusion was primarily one of a facilitator, intervening with measures aimed at increasing the employability particularly of the young and the long-term unemployed.

A Social Exclusion Unit was set up, reporting to the Prime Minister, to research into and produce 'joined up' inter-agency strategies for promoting **social inclusion**, as the right to participate in most aspects of social life, including work, education and leisure. Its remit covered groups such as teenage mothers, homeless people, and people living on poor council estates (Department of Social Security, 1999). Health Action Zones (HAZs) and Health Improvement Programmes (HIMPs) were established to develop local strategies for tackling inequalities in health, and were influenced by the same philosophy. Policies have therefore focused on local initiatives rather than national programmes of redistribution.

Thus the New Labour approach was one of enhancing equality of *opportunity*, rather than trying to equalise outcomes. In the words of Gordon Brown, as Chancellor of the Exchequer, the government rejected:

> equality of outcome not because it is too radical but because it is neither desirable nor feasible. (Brown, 1997, p. 19)

Underpinning this view is the belief that a strategy of merely increasing welfare benefits will serve only to compensate those in poverty without tackling the causes, while also serving to increase dependency and stifle human potential. However, the dilemma remains of how best to use benefits to alleviate poverty while waiting for social inclusion measures to take effect. It could take a very long time for opportunities to equalise!

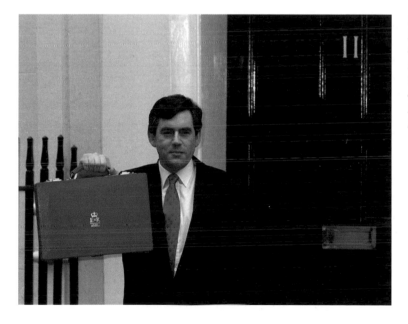

Chancellors of the Exchequer play a key role in defining poverty and in decisions that affect people's material circumstances. Here, Labour Chancellor Gordon Brown holds up the case containing his budget speech outside No. 11 Downing Street on 17 March 1998. (Photo: John Harris/Report Digital)

● What do you think is the advantage of social inclusion as an ideological framework for tackling poverty?

■ Social inclusion extends anti-poverty strategies from a concern with living standards to include a broader set of social rights of citizenship. It facilitates analysis of the obstacles involved in exclusion, and challenges society as a whole – not just governments – to develop appropriate measures that promote inclusion.

This approach also promotes an understanding of poverty and exclusion as something that is also experienced emotionally. In the words of Richard Wilkinson, a leading commentator on health inequalities:

> To feel depressed, cheated, bitter, desperate, vulnerable, frightened, angry, worried about debts or job and housing insecurity; to feel devalued, useless, helpless, uncared for, hopeless,

isolated, anxious and a failure: these feelings can dominate people's whole experience of life .... The material environment is merely the indelible mark and constant reminder of the oppressive fact of one's failure, of the atrophy of any sense of having a place in the community, and of one's social exclusion and devaluation as a human being. (Wilkinson, 1996, p. 215)

However, the strategy of social inclusion can be criticised not only for being insufficient, but also for having inherent dangers. For example, Ruth Lister (1998) has suggested that rather than social inclusion being seen as an integral part of a strategy to address material poverty, it has tended to supplant this and become the main goal in itself, particularly through inclusion in paid work. Far from addressing structural inequalities of income and wealth, the aim of getting people into jobs has taken over from the aim of abolishing poverty. The question has to be whether, in the context of entrenched structural inequalities, genuine social inclusion, including the eradication of poverty, is possible without greater equality (Lister, 1998, p. 224).

● What is a key disadvantage of identifying people as socially excluded?

■ Intentionally or otherwise, the rhetoric of social exclusion may stigmatise 'the poor' as a problematic group who refuse to join in. But this form of 'blaming the victim' further excludes people and can then be used to justify *enforced* participation.

The action of the Labour government of 1997 to retain the Job Seekers' Allowance placed an onus on unemployed claimants to prove that they were continuously seeking work. Additionally, the incentives to 'make work pay', e.g. through Working Families Tax Credit, led to a failure to improve the position of those on benefits for fear of reinforcing a dependency culture. Although the Labour government gave much greater priority to tackling poverty than previous Conservative governments had done, a 'strategy of inclusion' took priority over a 'strategy of equality', and the policy direction was clearly 'that wealth creation is now more important than wealth redistribution' (Steven Byers, Minister of Trade and Industry, cited in Watt *et al.*, 1999).

● Why would it be a mistake to equate paid work with social inclusion?

■ It does not recognise that those on benefits might seek other forms of participation (e.g. voluntary work), and that unpaid work, such as housework, child care and voluntary work, makes essential contributions to society.

The term **social capital** is used to describe the 'wealthiness' of communities whose assets include a wide range of features that together tend to affect the lives and health of the people who live in them. For example, systems of support and contact comprise a whole range of networks and involvement in a community, such as local school events, small pressure groups, the local theatre or sports groups, etc. From this contact, benefits accrue that result in a form of shared 'profit', which has become known as social capital.

However, the assets and profits of communities are not easily measured because they comprise a complex network of connections; this difficulty makes it harder to demonstrate that one of the benefits of increasing social capital is a reduction in inequalities in health. Nevertheless, Wilkinson (1996) has reviewed research that suggests communities with high social capital are less vulnerable to the direct material effects of poverty on health.[4]

9.6   Health or wealth?

9.6.1   Psychosocial effects of poverty

As we said at the beginning of this chapter, the relationship between poverty, exclusion and health is well established — people who are the most socially marginalized, such as unemployed people and those on low incomes, experience worse health than the general population. For example, they are more likely to live in overcrowded, damp and inadequately heated housing, which has a direct adverse effect on health, particularly among children.

However, an important element of research into inequalities in health that took place in the 1990s has been a shift of focus away from medical models that equate health with the absence of disease, towards social models that encompass physical, psychological and social well-being. Evidence is accumulating that attributes the risk to health associated with poverty and inequality not only to their **direct material effects,** e.g. insufficient money for a healthy diet, adequate heating and housing, etc., but also from the **psychosocial effects** of living in conditions of relative poverty.

This focus is evident in the proposition that social inclusion will protect health in two ways: first, indirectly through reducing the resort to health-damaging coping mechanisms, such as smoking and alcohol abuse; and second, more directly by acting on mind–body pathways to decrease vulnerability to mental and physical illness, for example by reducing mental stress that might otherwise lead to raised blood pressure and an increased risk of cardiovascular diseases (Chapter 8). This has led Richard Wilkinson to claim that:

> The social consequences of people's differing circumstances in terms of stress, self esteem and social relations may now be one of the most important influences on health. (Wilkinson, 1992, p. 168)

9.6.2   The Wilkinson hypothesis

One way of evaluating the psychosocial effects of poverty and social exclusion is to take a comparative approach to evidence from other countries, assessing whether health inequalities are indeed widest in societies where poverty and inequality is greatest. Figure 9.2 (*overleaf*) shows the results of one such study.

● Describe the patterns in the data in Figure 9.2 on the relationship between income and life expectancy.

■ There was a positive correlation between life expectancy at birth and income inequality in the countries selected for comparison. The countries with the lowest life expectancy (males and females combined) were those with the

[4] An extract, entitled 'The psychosocial causes of illness', from Richard Wilkinson's book *Unhealthy Societies: The Afflictions of Inequality* is reproduced in *Health and Disease: A Reader* (Open University Press, 3rd edn 2001), and is optional reading for Open University students studying this chapter.

Figure 9.2 *The cross-sectional relationship between income distribution and life expectancy (male and female combined) at birth in developed countries, around 1981. (Source: Wilkinson, R., 1996,* Unhealthy Societies: The Afflictions of Inequality, *Figure 5.3, p. 76.)*

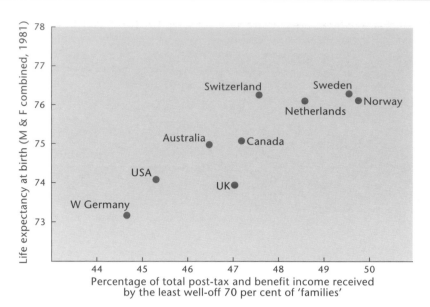

greatest relative poverty, defined as the share of income received by the least well-off 70 per cent of households. For example, in West Germany in 1981 the bottom 70 per cent of families who were least well off received only 44 per cent of the nation's post-tax and benefit income, and life expectancy at birth was only just above 73 years. Conversely, in Sweden and Norway the equivalent families received about 5 per cent more of the nation's income than in Germany, and life expectancy was about 3 years longer.

● What conclusions could be drawn from Figure 9.2 about the links between wealth distribution and health?

■ It is impossible to tell from these data whether there is a causal relationship between longevity and income inequality, but this research is consistent with the hypothesis that the more 'unequal' the distribution of wealth in a society, the greater the adverse effects on the health of the society *as a whole*.

This conclusion has become known as the **Wilkinson hypothesis** after its originator, who has assembled data to support it from many countries around the world. One example is Japan, where life expectancy at birth increased steadily over the same period in which income inequality decreased. The most controversial aspect of Wilkinson's research is that it leads to the inescapable conclusion that living in an unequal society damages the health of everyone, including those at the *top* of the income scale.

However, there are countries in Figure 9.2 that do not completely 'conform to type'; the UK was 'middling' in terms of income distribution, but did relatively poorly in terms of life expectancy. One explanation in terms of psychosocial effects on health might be that the nation's stock of social capital was low for reasons other than the extent of poverty.

When we relate the evidence on health (as expressed in terms of life expectancy) in Figure 9.2 to the level of national wealth in Table 9.5, there is no clear association. For example, the USA, West Germany and the UK were among the wealthiest countries in terms of total GDP (Table 9.5), yet did relatively poorly in terms of longevity (Figure 9.2).

Table 9.5 National wealth expressed as Gross Domestic Product (GDP) in US$, selected countries, 1980.

	Total GDP/US$ million	GDP per capita/US$
USA	216 881 467	111 804
Canada	2 671 923	111 131
Switzerland	691 539	101 891
Norway	381 867	9 510
Sweden	761 237	9 173
West Germany	5 471 383	8 891
Netherlands	1 231 162	8 704
Australia	1 241 702	8 486
United Kingdom	4 451 162	7 905

Source: Maddison, A. (1989) *The World Economy in the Twentieth Century*, OECD, Paris, p. 112.

● Does this analysis tend to support or undermine the Wilkinson hypothesis?

■ You might have agreed with Wilkinson's conclusion (1996) that in advanced industrialised countries, gross national wealth is less important to health than income distribution, and that the psychosocial effects of relative poverty are more important than levels of income themselves.

If this claim is correct (and the research is controversial), then policies that reduce social inequalities might have more effect on inequalities in health than could be achieved by putting more effort into increasing national wealth.

9.7 In conclusion

We began this book by stating that the greatest challenge to health-care provision was to be able to meet health needs within the available resources and in a way that upholds the key principles of the NHS. Fulfilling the principles of universality and accessibility is partly dependent upon how health care is defined. The strong association between inequalities in health and wealth presented in this and the previous chapter poses major dilemmas for policymakers, and indeed for all members of civil societies. To reduce social and economic inequality would require radical political and economic reforms, with far-reaching and unpredictable consequences, some of which may be undesirable to the majority. But perpetuating inequality is damaging not only to the health of people living in poverty, but may also have adverse effects on us all.

This observation has global as well as local relevance, as an article by D. R. Gwatkin, Director of the Health Policy Program at the World Bank, illustrates. It is called 'Health inequalities and the health of the poor. What do we know? What can we do?' (students of the Open University should read it now in *Health and Disease: A Reader* (Open University Press, 3rd edn 2001)). It reminds us that if we expand our gaze to reflect on the interaction of poverty, inequality, social exclusion and health in countries far beyond the UK, exactly the same issues and dilemmas apply.

OBJECTIVES FOR CHAPTER 9

9.1 Define and use, or recognise definitions and applications of, each of the terms printed in **bold** in the text.

9.2 Review alternative methods of defining poverty and comment on their implications for estimating the number of people living in poverty.

9.3 Discuss the causes of relative poverty in the UK in the twentieth century, illustrating the structural divisions in society and how they impact upon inequalities in health.

9.4 Critically discuss the ideologies that underpinned the anti-poverty strategies of successive UK governments from the 1960s to the end of the 1990s.

9.5 Describe hypotheses that link wealth, social exclusion and social capital to the health status of individuals and whole societies.

QUESTIONS FOR CHAPTER 9

1 (*Objective 9.2*)

In 1989, John Moore, who was then Secretary of State for Social Services, made the following assertion:

> ... by almost every material measure it is possible to contrive ... not only are those on lower incomes not getting any poorer, they are substantially better off than they ever were before. (Moore, 1989, p. 13)

What approach to defining poverty is implicit in this statement and on what grounds might it be criticised?

2 (*Objective 9.3*)

In 2000, the Health Secretary Alan Milburn focused his attention on ways of reducing the infant mortality rate (IMR). He concluded that:

> Major contributing factors are the child's birth weight, the mother's diet and her propensity to smoke. (*The Guardian*, 19 June 2000, p.19)

What does this focus on the individual behaviour of mothers fail to take into account in determining the underlying causes of infant mortality?

3 (*Objective 9.4*)

What similarities and what differences can you identify between the market approach to tackling poverty of the 1980s and early 1990s, and the social inclusion strategies introduced in 1997?

4 (*Objective 9.5*)

Explain how wealth might confer a health advantage on people who are better off, but at the same time lead to a reduction in health for society as a whole.

References and further sources

References

Abel-Smith, B. (1960) *A History of the Nursing Profession*, Heinemann, London.

Alaszewski, A. and Harvey, I. (2001) Health technology and knowledge; the creation and management of uncertainty and risk, in Davey, B. Gray, A. and Seale, C. (eds) *Health and Disease: A Reader*, 3rd edn, Open University Press, Buckingham.

Annandale, E. (1996) Working on the front-line: risk culture and nursing in the new NHS, *Sociological Review*, **44** (3), pp. 416–51.

Appleby, J. (1999) in Merry, P. (ed.) *Mellards NHS Handbook 1999/2000*, 14th edn, JMH Publishing, Kent.

Armstrong, D. (1995) The rise of surveillance medicine, *Sociology of Health and Illness*, **17** (3), pp. 393–404.

Atkinson, D. (1999) Research in practice, *Advocacy: A Review*, published for the Joseph Rowntree Foundation (York) by Pavilion Publishing, Brighton.

Austoker, J. (1990) *Breast Cancer Screening – Practical Guide for Primary Care Teams*, Cancer Research Campaign, London.

Baggott, R. (1998) *Health and Health Care in Britain*, Macmillan, Basingstoke.

Beck, U. (1992) *Risk Society: Towards a New Modernity*, Sage, London.

Bosma, H., Marmot, M. G., Hemingway, H. *et al.* (1997) Low job control and risk of coronary heart disease in the Whitehall II (prospective cohort) study, *British Medical Journal*, **314**, pp. 558–65.

Bowling, A. (1999) Ageism in cardiology, *British Medical Journal*, **319**, pp. 1353–5; also reproduced in Davey, B., Gray, A. and Seale, C. (eds) (2001) *Health and Disease: A Reader*, 3rd edn, Open University Press, Buckingham.

Bradshaw, A. (2000) Competence and British nursing: a view from history, *Journal of Clinical Nursing*, **9**, pp. 321–9.

British Medical Association (1999) *Withholding or Withdrawing Life-Prolonging Medical Treatment: Guidance for Decision-making*, BMJ Books, London.

Bunker, J.P. (1995) Medicine matters after all, *Journal of the Royal College of Physicians of London*, **29** (2), pp. 105–12. An edited extract also appears in Davey, B., Gray, A. and Seale, C. (eds) (2001) *Health and Disease: A Reader*, 3rd edn, Open University Press, Buckingham.

Burchill, F. and Casey, A. (1996) *Human Resource Management, the NHS: A case study*, Macmillan Business, Basingstoke and London.

Calman, K. (1999) Futures II, pp. 281–8 in Griffiths, S. and Hunter, J. (eds) *Perspectives on Public Health*, Radcliffe Medical Press, Oxford.

Cavelaars, A. E. J. M. *et al.* (2000) Educational differences in smoking: international comparison, *British Medical Journal*, **320**, pp. 1102–7.

Chandrasekar, C.R., Helliar, C.V., Lonie, A.A., Nixon, W.A. and Power, D.M. (1999) Strategic management of innovation risk in the biopharmaceutical industry: a UK perspective, *International Journal of Healthcare Technology and Management*, **1** (1/2), pp. 62–76.

Clegg, H. and Chester, T. (1957) *Wage Policy and the Health Service*, Basil Blackwell, Oxford.

Cowan, C. (2000) HCAs take a step nearer to join the club, *Nursing Times*, 13 April, **96**, No. 15.

Currie, G. (1999a) The influence of middle managers in the business planning process, *British Journal of Management*, **10** (2), pp. 141–156.

Currie, G. (1999b) The role of middle managers in strategic change: the emergence of a marketing strategy in a hospital trust, in Mark, A. and Dopson, S. (eds) *Organisational Behaviour in Health Care: The Future Research Agenda*, Macmillan, London.

Curtis Report (1946) *Report on the Care of Children*, Cmnd 6922, HMSO, London.

Davies, C. (1995) *Gender and the Professional Predicament in Nursing*, Open University Press, Buckingham; an edited version of the chapter, Professionalism and the conundrum of care, also appears in Davey, B., Gray, A. and Seale, C. (eds) (2001) *Health and Disease: A Reader*, 3rd edn, Open University Press, Buckingham.

Department of Health (1989) *Caring for People: Community Care in the Next Decade and Beyond*, HMSO, London.

Department of Health (1990) *NHS and Community Care Act*, HMSO, London.

Department of Health (1993) *Children First*, NHS Report No 9, HMSO, London.

Department of Health (1995) *The Carers (Recognition and Services) Act*, HMSO, London.

Department of Health (1997) *The New NHS Modern Dependable*, Cm. 3807, The Stationery Office, London.

Department of Health (1998a) *Modernising Social Services: Promoting Independence, Improving Protection, Raising Standards*, Cm. 4169, The Stationery Office, London.

Department of Health (1998b) *Partnership in Action: A Discussion Document*, The Stationery Office, London.

Department of Health (1999a) *Personal Social Services Current Expenditure in England, 1997-8*, Bulletin 1999/11, The Stationery Office, London.

Department of Health (1999b) *Community Care Statistics 1999: Home Help/Home Care Services, England*, The Stationery Office, London.

Department of Health (1999c) *NHS hospital and community health services non-medical staff in England: 1988–1998*, Statistical Bulletin 1999/12, The Stationery Office, London.

Department of Health (1999d) *Hospital, public health medicine and community health services medical and dental staff in England, 1988–1998*, Statistical Bulletin 1999/15, The Stationery Office, London.

Department of Health (1999e) *Research and Development in the Department of Health*, The Stationery Office, London; also available at www.doh.gov.uk/research, accessed 6 April 2001.

Department of Health (1999f) *Saving Lives: Our Healthier Nation*, Cm. 3852, The Stationery Office, London.

Department of Health (2000a) *The NHS Plan: A plan for investment*, Cm. 4818, The Stationery Office, London.

Department of Health (2000b) *Caring about Carers: National Strategy for Carers*, 2nd edn, The Stationery Office, London.

Department of Health (2000c) *Health and Personal Social Services Statistics*, www.doh.gov.uk, accessed May 2001.

Department of Health (2000d) *NHS hospital and community health services non-medical staff in England: 1989–1999*, Statistical Bulletin 2000/11,The Stationery Office, London.

Department of Health (2000e) *Hospital, public health medicine and community health services medical and dental staff in England, 1988–1998*, Statistical Bulletin 2000/9, The Stationery Office, London.

Department of Health (2000f) www.doh.gov.uk/wfprconsult, accessed 6 September 2000.

Department of Health (2000g) *Statistics for general medical practitioners in England: 1989–1999*, Statistical Bulletin 2000/0289, The Stationery Office, London; Statistical Press Release on www.doh.gov.uk accessed 6 September 2000.

Department of Health (2000h) *Research and Development for a First Class Service*, The Stationery Office, London.

Department of Health (2000i) *Coronary Heart Disease: National Service Framework*, The Stationery Office, London.

Department of Health (2000j) *Health Survey for England: The Health of Minority Ethnic Groups '99*, Volume 1, *Findings*, The Stationery Office, London.

Department of Health (2001a) *Inpatient and Outpatient Waiting in the NHS*, HC221, The Stationery Office, London.

Department of Health (2001b) www.doh.gov.uk/public/stats.3htm/

DHSS, London (1980) *Inequalities in Health*, Report of a Working Group (the 'Black Report'), Department of Health and Social Security.

Department of Health and Social Security (1989) *Working for Patients*, HMSO, London.

Department of Health and Social Services, Belfast (1997) *Well into 2000: a positive agenda for health and wellbeing*, The Stationery Office, Belfast; www.dhsspsni.gov.uk/publications/archived/well.htm, accessed on 11 October 2001.

Department of Social Security (1999) *Opportunity for All: Tackling Poverty and Social Exclusion*, The Stationery Office, London.

Doyal, L. and Cameron, A. (2001) Professions allied to medicine: continuity and change in a complex workforce, in Davey, B., Gray, A. and Seale, C. (eds) *Health and Disease: A Reader*, 3rd edn, Open University Press, Buckingham.

Doyal, L. and Pennell, I. (1979) *The Political Economy of Health*, Pluto Press, London.

Drever, F. and Whitehead, M. (1997) *Health Inequalities: Decennial Supplement*, DS Series no. 15, The Stationery Office, London.

Ebrahim, S. and Davey Smith, G. (2001) Multiple risk factor interventions for primary prevention of coronary heart disease (Cochrane Review), *The Cochrane Library*, Issue 3, 2001; abstract available at http://www.cochrane.org/cochrane/revabstr/ab001561.htm, accessed 12 October 2001.

Ebrahim, S., Davey Smith, G., McCabe, C. *et al.*, (1998) Cholesterol and coronary heart disease: screening and treatment, *Quality in Health Care*, **7**, pp. 232–9.

Edwards, N. (2000) Barrier relief, *Health Service Journal*, **110** (5698) 30 March, pp. 28–9.

Eurostat (1997) Income distribution and poverty in EU12 – 1993, *Statistics in Focus: Population and Social Conditions*, No. 6, Eurostat, Luxembourg.

Evans, M. (1998) Social security: dismantling the pyramids?, pp. 257–307 in Glennerster, H. and Hills, J. (eds) *The State of Welfare: The Economics of Social Spending*, Oxford University Press, Oxford.

Eysenbach, G., Ryoung Sa, E. and Diepgen, T.L. (2001) Towards the new millennium of cybermedicine, pp. 351–7 in Heller, T., Muston, R., Sidell, M. and Lloyd, C. (eds) *Working for Health*, Sage Publications, London.

Farmer, R. D. T. and Miller, D.L. (1983) *Lecture Notes on Epidemiology and Community Medicine*, Blackwell Scientific, Oxford.

Featherstone, M. and Hepworth, M. (1998) Ageing, the lifecourse and the sociology of embodiment, in Scambler, G. and Higgs, P. (eds) (1998) *Modernity, Medicine and Health*, Routledge, London.

Ferriman, A. (2000) Health and Social Services 'locked in a vicious cycle', *British Medical Journal*, **320**, p. 1692.

Frankel, S., Ebrahim, S. and Davey Smith, G. (2000) The limits to demand for health care, *British Medical Journal*, **321**, pp. 40–4.

Frayman, H. (1991) *Breadline Britain 1990s*, Domino Films/London Weekend Television, London.

Freund, P. E. S. and Maguire, M. B. (1995) *Health, Illness and the Social Body*, Prentice-Hall Inc., Englewood Cliffs, New Jersey.

Geissbuhler, V. and Eberhard, J. (2000) Waterbirths: a comparative study – a prospective study on more than 2 000 waterbirths, *Fetal Diagnosis and Therapy*, **15** (5), pp. 291-300.

George, V. and Wilding, P. (1999) *British Society and Social Welfare*, Macmillan, London.

Gordon, D. (2000) Inequalities in income, wealth and standard of living in Britain, pp. 25–58 in Pantazis, C. and Gordon, D. (eds) *Tackling Inequalities: Where Are We Now and What Can Be Done?*, Policy Press, Bristol.

Griffiths, R. (1983) *NHS Management Inquiry*, Department of Health and Social Security, London.

Grimshaw, J. M. and Russell, I. T. (1993) Effect of clinical guidelines on medical practice — a systematic review of rigorous evaluations, *Lancet*, **342** (8883), pp. 1317–22.

Gwatkin, D. R. (2000) Health inequalities and the health of the poor. What do we know? What can we do?, *Bulletin of the World Health Organization*, **78** (1), pp. 3-17; an edited extract also appears under the same title in Davey, B., Gray, A. and Seale, C. (2001) *Health and Disease: A Reader*, 3rd edn, Open University Press, Buckingham.

Hall, S. (1985) Religious ideologies and social movements in Jamaica, pp. 269–296 in Bocock, R. and Thompson, K. (eds) *Religion and Ideology: A Reader*, Manchester University Press, Manchester.

Ham, C. (1999) Improving NHS performance: human behaviour and health policy, first published in *British Medical Journal*, **319**, pp. 1490–2; an edited extract appears in Davey, B., Gray, A. and Seale, C. (eds) (2001) *Health and Disease: A Reader*, 3rd edn, Open University Press, Buckingham.

Ham, C. (2000) *The Politics of NHS Reform 1988–97*, King's Fund Publishing, London.

Hansard (House of Commons Parliamentary debates), 18 Jan 1983.

Hardey, M. (1998) Doctor in the house: The Internet as a source of lay health knowledge and the challenge to expertise, *Sociology of Health and Illness*, **21** (6), pp. 820–35, in *Communicating for Health: Working with Individuals and Groups*, The Open University. An edited extract appears in Davey, B., Gray, A. and Seale, C. (eds) (2001) *Health and Disease: A Reader*, 3rd edn, Open University Press, Buckingham.

Hardy, B. and Wistow, G. (1999) Changes in the private sector, in Hudson, B. (ed) *The Changing Role of Social Care*, Jessica Kingsley, London.

Harrison, A. and Prentice, S. (1996) *Acute Futures*, King's Fund Publishing, London.

Hattersley, L. (1999) Trends in life expectancy by social class — an update, *Health Statistics Quarterly*, **2**, pp. 16–24.

Health Services Journal (2000) editorial, p. 22.

Hemingway, H., Crook, A. M., Feder, G. *et al.* (2001) Underuse of coronary revascularization procedures in patients considered appropriate candidates for revascularization, *New England Journal of Medicine*, **344** (9), pp. 645–54.

Hills, J. (1998) *Income and Wealth: The latest evidence*, Joseph Rowntree Foundation, York.

Hippisley-Cox, J. and Pringle, M. (2001) General practice workload implications of the National Service Framework for coronary heart disease: cross-sectional survey, *British Medical Journal*, **323**, pp. 269–70.

Hippisley-Cox, J., Pringle, M., Crown, N., Meal, A. and Wynn, A. (2001) Sex inequalities in ischaemic heart disease in general practice: cross-sectional survey, *British Medical Journal*, **322**, p. 832.

House of Commons Health Committee (1991–2) *Second Report on Maternity Services* (the 'Winterton Report'), HMSO, London.

Human Fertilisation and Embryology Authority (2000) *Ninth Annual Report*, available from www.hfea.gov.uk, accessed 26 July 2001.

Hunt, C. (2000) Department of Health press release 2000/0463, 31 July 2000, www.doh.gov.uk.

Incomes Data Services (IDS) (1996) *Management Pay Review*, Issue 180, IDS London.

Jones, K., Brown, J. and Bradshaw, J. (1978) *Issues in Social Policy*, Routledge and Kegan Paul, London.

Joseph, K. and Sumption, J. (1979) *Equality*, J. Murray, London.

Klein, R. (1995) *The New Politics of the NHS*, Longman, Harlow.

Komaromy, C., Chant, L. and Sidell, M. (1999) *Better Health for Older People*, unpublished report, commissioned by the Health Education Authority.

Kuulasmaa, K., Tunstall-Pedoe, H., Dobson, A. *et al.* (2000) Estimation of contribution of changes in classic risk factors to trends in coronary-event rates across the WHO MONICA Project populations, *The Lancet*, **355**, pp. 675–87.

Lampe, F. C., Morris, R. W., Whincup, P. H. *et al.* (2001) Is the prevalence of coronary heart disease falling in British men? *Heart*, **8**, pp. 499–505.

Langlands, A. (1999) in *Department of Health Annual Report of the NHS Health Technology Assessment Programme*, The Stationery Office, London.

Langlands, A. (2000) *Department of Health – Research and Development for a First Class Service*, The Stationery Office, London.

Laupacis, A., Albers, G., Dalen, J., Dunn, M., Feinberg, W. and Jacobson, A. (1995) Antithrombotic therapy in atrial fibrillation, *Chest*, **108**, pp. 352–98.

Lawlor, D. A., Ebrahim, S. and Davey Smith, G. (2001) Sex matters: secular and geographical trends in sex differences in coronary heart disease mortality, *British Medical Journal*, **323**, pp. 541–5.

Lenaghan, J. (ed.) (1998) *Rethinking IT and Health*, Institute for Public Policy Research, London.

Lewis, J. and Piachaud, D. (1992) Women and poverty in the twentieth century, pp.27–45 in Glendinning, C. and Millar, J. (eds) *Women and Poverty in Britain: The 1990s*, Harvester Wheatsheaf, Hemel Hempstead.

Lip, G. Y. H. (1999) Thromboprophylaxis for atrial fibrillation, *The Lancet*, **353**, pp. 4–6.

Lister, R. (1998) From equality to social inclusion: New Labour and the welfare state, *Critical Social Policy*, **18** (2), pp. 215–25.

Low Pay Unit (1999) Creating a fairer Britain, *The New Review*, March/April, pp.16–8.

Mack, J. and Lansley, S. (1985) *Poor Britain*, Allen and Unwin, London. This work is updated in *Breadline Britain 1990s* (see Frayman, 1991).

MacPherson, S. and Silburn, R. (1998) The meaning and measurement of poverty, pp. 1–19 in Dixon, J. and Macarow, D. (eds) *Poverty: A Persistent Global Reality*, Routledge, London.

Maddison, A. (1989) *The World Economy in the Twentieth Century*, OECD, Paris.

Mahon, A. and Garrod, D. (2000) Fighting chance, *Health Service Journal*, **110** (5701), 20 April, pp. 26–27.

Manning, N. and Shaw, I. (1999) Mental health policy into the 21st century, *Policy and Politics*, **27** (1), pp. 5–12.

Marmot, M., Shipley, M., Brunner, E. and Hemingway, H. (2001) Relative contribution of early life and adult socioeconomic factors to adult morbidity in the Whitehall II study, *Journal of Epidemiology and Community Health*, **55**, pp. 301–7.

Marshall, K. (1996) Prevention. How much harm? How much benefit? *Canadian Medical Association Journal*, **155** (2), pp. 169–76; also reproduced in The Open University (2001) K203 *Working for Health*, Block 3, Unit 14.

Maynard, A. (1996) Evidence-based medicine: cost effectiveness and equity are ignored, *British Medical Journal*, **313**, p. 170. This letter is also reproduced in Davey, B., Gray, A. and Seale, C. (eds) (2001) *Health and Disease: A Reader*, 3rd edn, Open University Press, Buckingham.

McIntyre, A. (1998) Burden of illness review of obesity: are the true costs realised? *Journal of the Royal Society of Health*, **118**, pp. 76–84.

McKie, L. (1995) The art of surveillance or reasonable prevention: the case for cervical screening, *Sociology of Health and Illness*, **17** (4), pp. 441–57.

McPherson, K., Britton, A. and Causer, L. (2001) *Monitoring the progress of the 2010 target for coronary heart disease mortality: estimated consequences on CHD incidence and mortality from changing prevalence of risk factors* (A report for the Chief Medical Officer), London School of Hygiene and Tropical Medicine, in collaboration with the National Heart Forum.

Medical Devices Agency (2000) *Equipped to Care: The safe use of medical devices in the 21st century*, Medical Devices Agency, London.

Millar, J. and Glendinning, C. (1992) It all really starts in the home: gender divisions and poverty, pp. 3–10 in Glendinning, C. and Millar, J. (eds) *Women and Poverty in Britain: The 1990s*, Harvester Wheatsheaf, Hemel Hempstead.

Minghella, E., Ford, R., Freeman, T., Hoult, J., McGlynn, P. and O'Halloran, P. (1999) *Open All Hours: 24-hour response for people with mental health emergencies*, The Sainsbury Centre for Mental Health, London.

Modood, T., Berthoud, R., Lakey, J., Smith, P., Virdee, S. and Beishon, S. (1997) *Ethnic Minorities in Britain: Diversity and Disadvantage*, Policy Studies Institute, London.

Moody, A. (2001) Hospitals – who needs them?, Open University TV programme for U205 *Health and Disease*, and personal communication.

Moore, J. (1989) *The End of the Line for Poverty*, Conservative Political Centre, London.

Mulrow, C. (1987) The medical review article: state of the science, *Annals of Internal Medicine*, **166** (3), pp. 485–8.

New, B. (2000) An open debate is not an admission of failure (Commentary), *British Medical Journal*, **321**, p. 45.

New, B. (ed.) (1997) *Rationing: Talk and Action in Health Care*, British Medical Journal Publishing Group for The King's Fund, London.

New, B. and Mays, N. (1998) Age, renal replacement therapy and rationing, pp. 205–23 in *Health Care UK, 1996/97: The King's Fund review of health policy*, King's Fund Publishing, London.

NHS Executive (1999) *The Annual Report of the NHS Health Technology Assessment Programme*, Department of Health, London.

Nicholson, T. and Milne, R. (1999) *Beta interferons (1a and 1b) in relapsing-remitting and secondary progressive multiple sclerosis*, Development and Evaluation Committee Report No. 98, Wessex Institute for Health Research and Development, Southampton.

O'Brien, P. M., Wheeler, T. and Barker, D. J. (1999) Fetal programming: influences on development and disease in later life, *Proceedings of the 36th Royal College of Obstetricians and Gynaecologists' Study Group*, RCOG, London.

Office for National Statistics (1999) *New Earnings Survey 1999*, The Stationery Office, London.

Office for National Statistics (2000a) *Social Trends 30*, The Stationery Office, London.

Office for National Statistics (2000b) *Living in Britain: Results from the 1998 General Household Survey*, The Stationery Office, London.

Oppenheim, C. and Harker, L. (1996) *Poverty: The Facts*, Child Poverty Action Group, London.

Oxford Centre for Evidence-based Medicine (2001) Levels of evidence and grades of recommendation, http://www.jr2.ox.ac.uk/cebm/docs/levels.html; accessed 4 April 2001.

Parmanum, J., Field, D., Rennie, J. and Steer, P. (2000) National census of availability of neonatal intensive care, *British Medical Journal*, **321** (7263), pp. 727–9.

Petersen, S., Rayner, M. and Press, V. (2000) *Coronary Heart Disease Statistics: Annual Compendium 2000 edition*, British Heart Foundation Health Promotion Research Group, University of Oxford. Available online from: http://www.dphpc.ox.ac.uk/bhfhprg/stats/2000/index.html, accessed 17 October 2001.

Pollitt, C., Birchall, J. and Putman, K. (1998) *Decentralising Public Service Management*, Macmillan, Basingstoke.

Porte, M. (2000) *Health Service Journal*, The director's cut, 20 April, pp. 22–25.

Primatesta, P. and Poulter, N. R. (2000) Lipid concentrations and the use of lipid lowering drugs: evidence from a national cross sectional survey, *British Medical Journal*, **321**, pp. 1322-5.

Protheroe, J., Fahey, T., Montgomery, A. A. and Peters, T. J. (2000) The impact of patients' preferences on the treatment of atrial fibrillation: observational study of patient based decision analysis, *British Medical Journal*, **320**, pp. 1380–4.

RDSU Grants (1998) *Hit Rates of Different Funding Bodies* (http://www.rdsu.org.uk/geninfo/hitrate3.htm; accessed 6 September 2000)

Review Body for Nursing Staff, Midwives, Health Visitors and Professions Allied to Medicine (2000) *17th Report on Nursing Staff, Midwives and Health Visitors*, Cmnd 4563, The Stationery Office, London, pp. 55–6.

Roland, M. and Baker, R. (1999) *Clinical Governance: A Practical Guide for Primary Care Teams*, University of Manchester.

Rolph, S. (2000) *The history of community care in Norfolk 1930–1980: The role of two hostels*, unpublished PhD thesis, Open University.

Rosenthal, E. (1993) cited in Freund, P. E. S. and Maguire, M. G. (1995) *Health, Illness and the Social Body*, Prentice Hall Inc., Englewood Cliffs, New Jersey.

Royal College of Physicians (1991) *Preventive Medicine: A Report of a Working Party of the Royal College of Physicians*, RCP, London.

Royal Commission on Long-Term Care (1999) *With Respect to Old Age. Long-term Care – Rights and Responsibilities*, Cmnd 4192, The Stationery Office, London.

Sackett, D. L., Rosenberg, W. M. C., Gray, J. A. M. and Haynes, R. B. (1996) Evidence-based medicine: what it is and what it isn't, *British Medical Journal*, **312**, pp. 71–2. This article is also reproduced in Davey, B., Gray, A. and Seale, C. (eds) (2001) *Health and Disease: A Reader*, 3rd edn, Open University Press, Buckingham.

Salvage, J. (1985) *The Politics of Nursing*, Heinemann Nursing, London.

Scottish Office (1999) *Towards a Healthier Scotland: A White Paper on Health*, HMSO, Edinburgh, Cmnd 4269; http://www.scotland.gov.uk/library/documents-w7/tahs-00.htm, accessed 12 October 2001.

Scottish Office Department of Health (1998) *Working Together for a Healthier Scotland: a consultation document*, The Stationery Office, Edinburgh.

Secretary of State for Wales (1998) *Better health, better Wales: a consultative paper*, Welsh Office, Cardiff.

Shaw, M., Dorling, D., Gordon, D. and Davey Smith, G. (1999) *The Widening Gap: Health Inequalities and Policy in Britain*, Policy Press, Bristol.

Shiu, M. (1993) Refusing to treat smokers is unethical and a dangerous precedent, *British Medical Journal*, **306**, pp. 1048–9; also reproduced in Davey, B., Gray, A. and Seale, C. (eds) (2001) *Health and Disease: A Reader*, 3rd edn, Open University Press, Buckingham.

Social Services Inspectorate (1998) *Moving into the Mainstream: Inspection of Services for Adults with Learning Disabilities*, Department of Health, London.

Social Services Select Committee (1985) *Community Care with Special Reference to Adult Mentally Ill and Mentally Handicapped People*, HMSO, London.

Stacey, M. (1969) The myth of community studies, *British Journal of Sociology*, **20** (2), pp. 134–47.

Stacey, M. (1991) *The Sociology of Health and Healing: A Textbook*, Routledge, London and New York.

Strauss, A., Schatzman, L., Ehrlich, D., Bucher, R. and Sabshin, M. (1963) The hospital and its negotiated order, in Friedson, E., Salaman, G. and Thompson, K. (eds) *People and Organisations*, Longman, London.

Strong, P. and Robinson, J. (1988) *New Model Management: Griffiths and the NHS*, Nursing Policy Studies Centre, Warwick.

The Open University (1983) *D208: Decision making in Britain*, Open University Press, Buckingham.

The UK Renal Registry (1999) *The Second Annual Report – December 1999*, The UK Renal Registry, Bristol.

Thornley, C. (1996a) Segmentation and inequality in the nursing workforce: reevaluating the evaluation of skills, in Crompton, R., Gallie, D. and Purcell, K. (eds) *Changing Forms of Employment: Organisations, Skills and Gender*, Routledge, London and New York.

Thornley, C. (1996b) *Dispelling the Myth: Nursing Pay Trends 1979–1996*, UNISON, London.

Thornley, C. (1997) *The Invisible Workers: An Investigation into the Pay and Employment of Health Care Assistants in the NHS*, UNISON, London, pp. 1–22.

Thornley, C. (1998a) *A Question of Fairness: Nurses' pay trends 1979–96*, UNISON, London.

Thornley, C. (1998b) Contesting local pay: The decentralisation of collective bargaining in the NHS, *British Journal of Industrial Relations*, **36** (3), pp. 413–434.

Thornley, C. (1998c) *Neglected Nurses, Hidden Work: An investigation into the pay and employment of nursing auxiliaries/assistants in the NHS*, UNISON, London, pp. 1–52.

Thornley, C. (1999) *Out of Sight, Out of Mind: Evidence and Perspectives on the Recruitment and Retention of Non-Registered Nursing Staff in the NHS*, UNISON, London, pp. 5–26.

Tones, K. (1993) Radicalism and the ideology of health education, *Health Education Research*, **8** (2), pp. 147–50.

Toop, L. and Richards, D. (2001) Preventing cardiovascular disease in primary care (editorial), *British Medical Journal*, **323**, pp. 246–7.

Townsend, P. (1979) *Poverty in the United Kingdom*, Allen Lane and Penguin, University of California Press, London and Berkeley, CA.

Traynor, M. (1999) *Managerialism and Nursing: Beyond Oppression and Profession*, Routledge, London.

Tunstall-Pedoe, H., Kuulasmaa, K., Mahonen, M. *et al.* (1999) Contribution of trends in survival and coronary-event rates to changes in coronary heart disease mortality: 10-year results from 37 WHO MONICA Project populations, *The Lancet*, **353**, pp. 1547–57.

Underwood, M. J. and Bailey, J. S. (1993) Coronary bypass surgery should not be offered to smokers, *British Medical Journal*, **306**, pp. 1047–8; also reproduced in Davey, B., Gray, A. and Seale, C. (eds) (2001) *Health and Disease: A Reader*, 3rd edn, Open University Press, Buckingham.

van Rossum, C. T. M., Shipley, M. J., van de Mheen, H., Grobbee, D. E. and Marmot, M. G. (2000) Employment grade differences in cause specific mortality. A 25 year follow up of civil servants from the first Whitehall study, *Journal of Epidemiology and Community Health*, **54**, pp. 178–84.

Wallace, S. (1998) Telemedicine in the NHS for the Millennium and Beyond, pp. 55–100 in Lenaghan, J. (ed.) *Rethinking IT and Health*, Institute for Public Policy Research, London.

Warner, L. and Wexler, S. (1998) *Eight hours a day and taken for granted*, The Princess Royal Trust for Carers, London.

Watt, N., Hencke, D. and Gow, D. (1999) 'Wealth creation is the priority', insists minister, *The Guardian*, 3 February.

Wild, S. and McKeigue, P. (1997) Cross-sectional analysis of mortality by country of birth in England and Wales 1970–92, *British Medical Journal*, **314**, pp. 705–10.

Wilkinson, R. (1992) Income distribution and life expectancy, *British Medical Journal*, **304**, pp. 165–8.

Wilkinson, R. (1996) *Unhealthy Societies: The Afflictions of Inequality*, Routledge, London and New York; an edited extract, The psychosocial causes of illness, also appears in Davey, B., Gray, A. and Seale, C. (2001) *Health and Disease: A Reader*, 3rd edn, Open University Press, Buckingham.

Williams, A. (1996) QALYS and ethics: A health economist's perspective, *Social Science and Medicine*, **43**, pp. 1795–1804.

Williams, A. (1997a) How should information on cost effectiveness influence clinical practice? in Culyer, A. J. and Maynard, A. K. (eds) *Being Reasonable about the Economics of Health*, Edward Elgar, Cheltenham.

Williams, A. (1997b) Priority setting in public and private health care: A guide through the ideological jungle, in Culyer, A. J. and Maynard, A. K. (eds) *Being Reasonable about the Economics of Health*, Edward Elgar, Cheltenham.

Wilson, J. M. G. and Jungner, S. (1968) *The Principles and Practice of Screening for Disease*, Public Health Papers 34, World Health Organisation, Geneva.

World Health Organisation (2000) *Health Systems: Improving Performance*, World Health Organisation, Geneva.

Wyke, S., Myles, S. and Popay J. (1999) Total purchasing, community and continuing care, *Health and Social Care in the Community*, **7** (6), pp. 394–407.

Further Sources

Chapter 2

Drummond, M. F. *et al.* (1997) *Methods for the Economic Evaluation of Health Care Programmes*, 2nd edn, Oxford University Press, Oxford, especially Ch. 6, pp. 139–83.

Edwards, R. T. (1997) *NHS Waiting Lists: Towards the Elusive Solution*, Office of Health Economics, London, has a fuller discussion of the waiting list phenomenon.

McGuire, A., Henderson, J. and Mooney, G. (1988) *The Economics of Health Care*, Routledge and Kegan Paul, London.

Chapter 3

If you want to follow up topical issues in the rapidly changing world of NHS management, then the weekly *Health Service Journal* published every Thursday is an invaluable guide. As well as topical reporting and editorial and views from NHS staff and managers, it includes brief summaries of relevant academic research.

Clarke, J. (ed.) (2001) *New Managerialism, New Welfare?* Open University Press, Buckingham. This textbook provides a useful overview of how the development of managerialism has affected welfare policy and delivery under Labour governments. It includes two specific chapters on health care, and explores how the New Labour version of managerialism impacts on all sectors of social welfare.

Exworthy, M. and Halford, S. (eds) (1999) *Professionals and the New Managerialism*, Open University Press, Buckingham, contains a series of articles exploring the way in which managerialism interacts with the lives of health professionals.

Harrison, S. and Pollitt, C. (1994) *Controlling Health Professionals*, Open University Press, Buckingham, is a fascinating exploration of how governments try to maintain a degree of control over health services.

Strong, P and Robinson, J. (1990) *The NHS Under New Management*, Open University Press, Buckingham, an excellent study of how early managerial reforms were introduced into the NHS in the 1980s, has become a sociological classic and is a thoroughly enjoyable and humane book to read.

Chapter 4

Brechin, A., Walmsley, J., Katz, J. and Peace, S. (1998) *Care Matters: concepts, practice and research in health and social care*, Sage Publications, London, Thousand Oaks, New Delhi. A team of lecturers at The Open University has written a book that draws upon a range of academic disciplines to provide a shared meaning of the concept of care. They highlight the balance between independence, interdependency and dependency.

Hogg, C. (1999) *Patients, Power and Politics: from patients to citizens*, Sage Publications, London, Thousand Oaks, New Delhi. The involvement of users in health care is an important area of concern. This book highlights how individuals as patients, healthy people and research subjects relate to health services.

Stacey, M. (1999) *The Sociology of Health and Healing*, Routledge, London and New York. This textbook provides a historical approach to health and healing and a sociological analysis of the division of labour and concepts of health and illness, and puts 'caring' into a broader context.

Chapter 5

Abel-Smith, B. (1960) *A History of the Nursing Profession*, Heinemann. The classic history of the nursing profession and still a great read. The book lays bare the issues of status and hierarchy, and explores employer and union/association strategy on training, pay and conditions in the formalisation of nursing from the early 19th century onwards.

Davies, C. (1995) *Gender and the Professional Predicament in Nursing*, Open University Press, Buckingham. A brave and direct focus on gender, and analysis of problems with gendered conceptualisations of skills and professionalism. One of the key debates for the 21st century.

Doyal, L. and Pennell, I. (1979) *The Political Economy of Health*, Pluto Press, London. Still a path-breaking book which employs a politico-economic and internationalist approach to the analysis of ill health and disease and the health division of labour.

Stacey, M. (1991) *The Sociology of Health and Healing: A Textbook*, Unwin Hyman London. A wealth of rich detail and history in a strongly theoretical sociological approach, where the division of labour, especially as it relates to class and gender, is viewed as central.

Thornley, C., Ironside, M. and Seifert, R. (2000) UNISON and changes in collective bargaining in health and local government, in Terry, M. (ed.) *Redefining Public Service Unionism*, Routledge, London and New York. For readers unfamiliar with the industrial relations discipline, this chapter offers a concise and up-to-date introduction to the key issues for health-service workers and their representative organisations for the early years of the 21st century. It explores in particular the challenges for UNISON, the largest trade union in the NHS (and in the UK).

Chapter 6

An interesting arena of sociological debate on research methods can be found in Hammersley, M. and Gomm, R. (1997) *Bias in Social Research Online*, **2** (1), http://www.socresonline.org.uk/socresonline/2/1.html

Berg, M. and Mol, A. (eds) (1998) *Differences in Medicine*, Duke University Press, Durham and London, brings together interdisciplinary and intercultural ideas that challenge conventional, Western, medical wisdom.

Potter, J. (1996) *Representing Reality: Discourse, Rhetoric and Social Construction*, Sage Publications, London. Broader challenges to the way that evidence is constructed and the way that we think about facts are presented in this book.

Chapter 7

Beck, U. (1992) *Risk Society: Towards a New Modernity*, Sage Publications, London. Considered to be a core sociological text, particularly relevant in its discussion of risk in society. It moves beyond health to consider how society's focus on risk from the late twentieth century has shaped the way we live. This book provides an interesting foundation for some of the ideas introduced in Chapter 7 that relate to risk and medical technology.

Freund, P. E. S. and McGuire, M. G. (1995) *Health, Illness and the Social Body*, Prentice Hall, Englewood Cliffs, New Jersey. Chapter 7 has touched on some ideas developed in the discipline of medical sociology, and this book is suitable for students wishing to read further on this topic. Its main focus is on the relationships of power in health and illness.

Lenaghan, J. (ed.) (1998) *Rethinking IT and Health*, Institute for Public Policy Research, London. The rate of change in the UK health-care system since the 1980s has been rapid and is ongoing. Information and communication are at the centre of these changes and this book brings together a collection of writings by six authors with specialist knowledge in this area. The book editor, Jo Lenaghan, has an interest in patient rights within health care.

Chapter 8

Heller, T., Muston, R., Sidell, M. and Lloyd, C. (eds) (2001) *Working for Health*, Sage Publications, London, is a collection of contributions from different disciplines that conveys dynamic accounts of health. These include theory and ideology, social patterns of health, public health issues and individual accounts of health, caring and curing.

Griffiths, S. and Hunter, D. J. (eds) (1999) *Perspectives in Public Health*, Radcliffe Medical Press, Oxford, brings together a review of the policy and practice in public health.

Statistics on CHD mortality, morbidity and costs can be found at: http://www.dphpc.ox.ac.uk/bhfhprg/stats/2000/2000/pdf/2000stats.pdf

Tones, B. K. (1992) Health promotion, empowerment and the concept of control, in *Health Education: Politics and Practice*, Deakin University Press, Victoria, presents a fuller discussion of health education as empowerment.

Chapter 9

Bartley, M., Blane, D. and Davey-Smith, G. (eds) (1998) *The Sociology of Health Inequalities*, Blackwell Publishers, Oxford, puts together a range of articles that help to provide insights into some of the fine grain of inequalities in health from a sociological perspective. They make links between individual behaviour and social structure and include articles that debate issues in men's health, genetics and ethnicity and in geography and health inequalities.

Townsend, P., Davidson, N and Whitehead, M. (eds) (1988) *The Health Divide*, Penguin, England, combines in a single volume two classic texts for understanding inequalities in health (the Black Report).

Answers to questions

Chapter 1

1 You might have included some of the following points in your answer:

- Politicians have to balance the competing demands for NHS resources in an equitable way, while at the same time trying to retain or secure their popularity with the electorate.

- If governments were to respond to such demands by increasing resources to NICUs, it might open the floodgates to other equally worthy and publicly appealing needs.

- Given that resources are finite, any increase in one area of care inevitably results in a reduction in health-care provision elsewhere. Who would decide where the cuts would fall?

2 The answer to this question depends upon how benefit is defined and also the timescale in which any evaluation is made. There are both short- and long-term outcomes of neonatal intensive care. But when the number of available NICU cots is limited, difficult choices have to be made about whether or not to treat babies whose chances of survival are very low. It follows that there is a strong case for making judgements on the benefits and drawbacks of neonatal intensive-care treatments.

It could be argued that it is better to treat all babies who need intensive care, even when their prognosis is poor, because all life is sacred so every attempt must be made to sustain life. Indeed, some parents might argue that a short life afforded to their baby is better than no life at all and that grief is made more bearable by the knowledge that everything has been done to try to save their baby's life. You might have also presented the opposing ethical view that the amount of intervention required in supporting the lives of very sick and premature babies cannot be justified ethically, because the extensive resources required to 'rescue' them might have saved more lives if allocated elsewhere, or because the quality of the babies' lives is likely to be very poor.

Chapter 2

1 You might have pointed out that the tight structuring and management of consultation time meant that more people could be seen in the clinic. This is one form of allocative efficiency and you could have argued that, on balance, the individual costs for Rosie of waiting were outweighed by the benefit of many more people being seen at the clinic. You might also have suggested that this case study raised other opportunity costs. For example, there is the time and distress that Rosie experienced during her wait for the appointment, which was not relieved by seeing the consultant. Rosie then had to face a further period of waiting in uncertainty for the diagnostic test and possibly further waits if the result was inconclusive. By not giving Rosie the full opportunity to describe her symptoms and raise her concerns, the consultant might have missed important information that could have indicated the need for a different form of investigation. The consultant might also have been able to reduce Rosie's level of anxiety. The 'technical' efficiency of the clinic appointment system could be a short-term saving with a long-term cost. It raises the dilemma of how to allocate the 'appropriate' amount of time to people when there is not enough of the health-care professionals' time to go around and when the focus is upon reducing waiting list times.

2   One of the dilemmas is how to allocate resources in an efficient and equitable way when it is difficult to predict the extent of the need. Even if the solution of keeping some spare capacity is used, then it is still impossible to predict how much will be needed. While some surgery is known to require ITU post-operative support so that some ITU needs are predictable, many of the beds are taken up by unpredictable emergency referrals. This example also raises the issue of how to allocate resources according to the best outcome for patients. Hannah had a better chance of recovery than Ben, but how could the choice be made? The criteria used to allocate beds do not allow for the difficulty of being unable to predict outcomes. Regardless of the rationing mechanisms that exist for allocating health-care services, these sorts of dilemma remain.

3   You might have made the general point that efficiency measures do not really resolve the dilemma of equalising inequalities and improving the health of the most 'unhealthy' people in society. There is a trade-off between equity and efficiency that involves complex decisions and raises the question of whose values should count most. The inevitable outcome is that any attempt to reduce inequalities involves some form of discrimination. You might also have stated that the quality of the information that informs decision-making influences the process, and therefore is very significant. However, there are other factors, such as economic, political, ideological and ethical ones, that impact upon the ways in which health care is delivered,

Chapter 3

1   You might have suggested that the main difficulties lie in the balance between delegation and control. The extent to which governments (at the centre) allow local managers to use their own leadership skills has varied over time and is constrained by political and economic directives. Clinical decision-making in the NHS takes place locally and is dependent upon medical expertise. This creates a further territorial tension between central and local managers and clinicians. When clinicians are also managers, the relationships are further complicated.

2   (a) Pauline has to face the conflict between her role as the patients' advocate and her role as budget manager. How can she manage the constraints of the staff budget when patient care might be compromised? She is directly responsible for the nursing care of patients during their stay on the ward and she must decide what constitutes safe practice, but it is difficult for her to oppose the surgeon, who appears to have support from hospital managers. Furthermore, Pauline needs to be supported by her staff, who will resent any demands to compromise the care that they give to their patients. They might also feel betrayed by Pauline's apparent loyalty to 'management' above the needs of 'her' patients and staff.

   (b) You might have suggested that giving poorer quality care could be more costly in the long term. For example, patients' recovery might be affected, thus prolonging their stay, or they might have to be readmitted.

   (c) The chapter makes the point that doctors as managers wield more power because they are also clinicians and benefit from this higher status, whereas nurses in their managerial role experience relatively more isolation from their colleagues in a profession that has traditionally been more collective than medicine. Both doctors and nurses experience a conflict of role and identity that arises from their need to serve the best interests of their patients and to impose resource constraints on health-care delivery. However, nurses do not have the same level of independence as doctors, who are part of a well-protected professional group. In particular, senior doctors also have a higher degree of financial independence.

3   In primary care, GPs act as independent contractors to the NHS, but the growth of PCTs changes their identity from local doctor to large-scale health-care commissioner. The role involves complex and time-consuming activities, which potentially reduces their time for their clinical practice. More than this, it is predicted to impact detrimentally upon the doctor–patient relationship, and the dual role could result in an erosion of trust between them through their conflicting interests. Conversely, the increased power of PCTs could tip the balance of power from tertiary to primary care, and increase patient trust. This is particularly so with the increased number of GPs in each Trust and their subsequent removal from direct managerial responsibility.

Chapter 4

1   Care in the community remains dependent upon care by informal carers. Although Lucy's needs are relatively small, the trend in the reduction of domestic and formal social care suggests that she will not get the support she needs to enable her to stay at home. Not providing a low level of care to enable people to retain some degree of independence could be a false economy in the longer term. People who become dependent are more likely to develop escalating care needs.

2   The term 'community care' has been the focus of sociological debate and it has been concluded that it is not only unhelpful but potentially dangerous. This is because it is prescriptive and reinforces the burden of care for the family, and in particular the expectation for women to be carers. The term 'care' places expectations of care upon informal carers through an assumed duty to 'be caring'. Formal carers have to wrestle with the distinctions between health-care and social-care needs and manage joined-up working.

3   Sally's needs for autonomy conflict with the need for her formal carers to keep her 'safe' from harm. Furthermore, her formal carers are responsible for ensuring that, if Sally does not abide by the conditions of her care plan, under the 1996 Mental Health (Patients in the Community) Act, she would be forced to take her medication. The dilemma here is how to protect the rights of mental health patients such as Sally, including the right to refuse treatment, when people with concerns for public safety believe that compulsory treatment in the community is the only way to achieve this.

You might have gone on to say that people with mental health needs often suffer from the stigma associated with mental illness that constructs them as dangerous. The rights of users of mental health services to live in the community can conflict with the rights of the public to be protected from harm, and this conflict acts against community integration and support. The revolving door of emergency admissions remains a feature of the life of many people with mental health needs.

Chapter 5

1   In this labour-intensive sector, cost-restraint strategies based on narrow conceptions of efficiency tend to focus on ways of restraining the paybill. In the chapter, you have seen both the historical and the modern use of the methods of:

   (a) manipulation of pay determination processes and outcomes;

   (b) manipulation of grademix (labour substitution);

   (c) workload increases.

   However, each method tends to run into problems of equity and efficiency, problems that were illustrated in case study of HCAs in the NHS.

2   You will probably have found that there is no easy answer to this apparently simple question! Some clues are to be found in the historical roots of the modern division of health-care labour, where early gender (and class) divisions in the wider economy and society were highly influential. The early formalisation of health-care provision thus proceeded along gendered lines, with male doctors quickly establishing formal mechanisms of power and control within the health hierarchy (not least through the formation of professional associations and measures taken to restrict labour supply), and for some time excluding women from medical occupations altogether. The attempt by women to form a 'profession' for themselves in reaction to this can be seen as highly influential in the early development of nursing (and PAMs), and is still visible in modern nurse 'professionalising' strategies.

   How much has changed? Women fought both individually and collectively to be allowed into the medical profession and you saw that the 1990s produced an increase in the proportion of women doctors. However, three factors may make progress slow:

   (a) Women are still disproportionately constrained by their dual domestic and work roles — the 'long hours' culture of many male-dominated professions like medicine tends to militate against this combination of roles by women who still perform the great majority of housework and informal caring work within the home and community.

   (b) There may still be some very strong resistance within the medical (and other) professions to women's entry and progression up the career hierarchy, particularly where this is seen to challenge male authority and comfort both at work and in the home. This resistance may be hard to counter through legislative and policy means.

   (c) Women themselves may not wish to compete on male territory in jobs largely organised along gendered lines, but may alternatively seek to gain full recognition and reward for the jobs they already do (as in the case of HCAs and NAs).

3   You probably had mixed views on how to answer this question. On the one hand, the rationale for 'professionalisation' can be understood in the light of the broader division of health-care labour, including gender issues: some degree of success could be claimed in the fact of nurse registration itself, and in an increasing emphasis historically on academic training and qualifications, and eventually pay. They have succeeded in gaining new top posts for nurses,

such as nurse consultants. On the other hand, you have also seen that, as nurses' pay rose, employer strategies have historically focused on substituting cheaper labour for registered nurses, particularly at times of shortages. These strategies have been conducted with relative ease, made possible by the difficulty of defining 'care work' itself and who should do what. Celia Davies, Lesley Doyal and Ann Bradshaw agree that these dilemmas for employee strategy are likely to be the subject of debate for some time.

4   You saw from the case study that it has always been inappropriate to describe NAs as 'unskilled' workers, and that both they and the new grade of HCAs gain a high degree of knowledge through informal care-work and experiential (on-the-job) learning, to the extent that most argue they regularly substitute for registered nursing staff on the wards and in the community. It is also increasingly inappropriate to describe either group as 'unqualified' – many have gained or are in the process of gaining NVQs. These qualifications are providing a system of accreditation that might start to run in parallel to registered-nurse training as well as already leading into it.

Given this context, it is difficult to account for the pay and conditions of HCAs being worse than those for NAs as their roles are virtually identical. Here, we probably need to look to the role of *local* pay determination for HCAs in undermining *national* rates for NAs, and it is interesting to speculate on the extent to which this was always a desired outcome of employer strategy. This apparent inequity is compounded by a further one, i.e. the fact that the work already performed by NAs was undervalued, shown in part by the widening differentials between NAs and registered nurses over the past two decades. In this respect, recent research into the roles of HCAs also raises wider dilemmas around pay and grademix within nursing, as opposed to between nursing and other health occupations.

Chapter 6

1   There is an assumption that decision-makers will be able to agree on what the problem is that is being considered. Apart from research evidence being perceived to be of a sufficiently good quality, it also needs to address the right question. An important part of evaluating evidence is to check whether the research under scrutiny has asked the most appropriate question in order to produce the information that is needed. In part this is dependent upon an agreement being reached between interested parties, including potential funders, in the research development process (step 1).

It is also assumed that decision-makers, particularly those from different disciplines who often have competing interests, will be in agreement about the desired outcomes of decisions.

Step 3 of the rational model assumes that an agreement can be reached about what constitutes a sufficient amount of evidence, when in reality to list all the various ways of achieving outcomes is a potentially endless task! Finally, there is an assumption that it will be possible to recognise and agree on the 'best' way when there could be several equally valid possibilities from which to choose, or no obvious 'best' way. Therefore, a useful question to ask when assessing evaluation evidence is 'What criteria were used to assess the evidence?'

2   In your answer, you might have included the questions similar to the following.

- How many people were there in each group in the trial?
- How representative of the population as a whole or of depressed people was each sample group?
- What were the completion rates of the interventions?
- How were the participants recruited to the trial?
- What they were told about their participation in the study?
- Were the members of each group treated in the same hospital or clinic?

3   You might have suggested the following points.

RCTs are not suitable for all forms of evaluation. They are very expensive and time-consuming, and they need to enrol a large number of 'subjects' into the trials; more significantly perhaps, they are limited in what they can measure. Furthermore, opportunity costs and quality-of-life measurements are not always taken into account in efficiency evaluations. The take-up of treatment interventions is dependent upon a clear understanding of the needs of patients, and yet often they are involved in decision-making only at the point of choosing from a selection of treatments. The ways in which patients make treatment decisions are much more suited to qualitative studies.

RCTs are also notoriously poor measures of comparisons between large groups, such as clinical departments, and larger organisations, such as hospitals, because they need large numbers of each unit of study to be entered into the trial. Without large numbers, randomising into two groups will not produce comparability between them, nor will it be possible to generalise to a wider population.

4   It is most likely that medical decision-makers will have been socialised into a culture in which the scientific paradigm dominates, and therefore will be most strongly influenced by 'gold standard' research findings. Conversely, local research findings that are seen to be appropriate for particular settings will stand a greater chance of being translated into practice. The take-up of treatment options that 'experts' consider to be effective will be lower when they conflict with the wishes of individual patients.

Despite the legal requirement to respect patient autonomy, and the discrepancy between the needs of patients and expert opinion, there is a paucity of research into the criteria by which patients make decisions. Research into the decision-making process using qualitative data or a multi-method approach is more likely to contribute to the type of evidence that takes into account the patient's/ user's perspective in a meaningful way. David Sackett would argue that patient choice should be part of the research process.

Chapter 7

1   You might have referred back to Chapter 6, which raised some of the difficulties in the evaluation of health-care innovations. It is important to know not only which technologies work effectively but also what harmful effects there might be, and safety is a significant concern for governments. The process of evaluating the long-term effects of any intervention makes the development and evaluation long and costly. Even with cost and safety controls in place, there will be many more cost-effective and safe treatments available than can be afforded in the NHS budget, and choices have to be made about which to use. How

governments choose between equally worthy alternatives is one of the key dilemmas in UK health care.

2   IVF is both a product and a process innovation. You might have argued that the technological imperative helps to explain the development of IVF, in which the boundaries of what it is possible to do have been pushed back. Certainly IVF has quickly become a routine treatment for infertility. However, this explanation is limited by factors such as the trend towards later reproduction by many families and the subsequent increased demands for a technological solution to the problem for some people of failure to conceive, especially when there is a limited time before fertility reduces dramatically. Therefore the technological imperative drives what it is possible to do, and is driven by the need for change.

3   You may well have qualified this statement by questioning the context. For example, what is health care and where is it given? If it is taken as formal health care, then the potential for increased choice is made greater by medical innovations. One example is that of being able to manage one's own care at home instead of needing to stay in hospital, and you might have cited the case of renal dialysis. If health care includes informal care too, then there has been a comparatively lower investment in providing support to informal carers and their situations, as discussed in Chapter 4. People who use complementary therapies, or are interested in accessing medical information to help with decisions about health care, will probably benefit from E-health. However, all of these examples are constrained by the fact that there are gatekeepers, most commonly GPs who manage access to formal and free-at-source health care. This means that those people in society who are most aware and most articulate are more likely to influence access to health resources than people who are less knowledgeable about what is available, with limited access to resources.

4   MRI is a good example of an innovation that can reduce the risk of existing visualising technologies. You might have stated that this development was not directly planned and evolved along an incremental route. There were several groups of people working in many different ways with the associated technologies, and the medical application was a small part of this. Thus, the comparative safety of MRI was secondary to its multidisciplinary development process. Interestingly with MRI, its application has been more driven by 'other' capacities than safety, most particularly the accuracy and detail of the information that is produced by the scans. For example, the fact that MRI has the capacity to provide information that would otherwise be provided by several different and invasive techniques seems to have taken second place to considerations of cost, which might be a false economy in the long term. In the TV programme, Alan Moody makes the point that MRI is used as a *last* rather than a *first* resort.

Chapter 8

1   Hip-replacement surgery is an example of tertiary prevention, because this treatment aims to reduce the pain and immobility caused by the arthritic hip.

Anti-pollution legislation is a health-protection measure contributing to both primary and secondary prevention: it aims to prevent the development of respiratory illness in people who have not yet been affected (primary prevention), and reduce the adverse effects of pollution on those who already have a sensitivity to smoke pollution (secondary prevention).

Warnings about poor air quality are a health-education measure aimed at people who are already vulnerable to the effects of atmospheric pollution (secondary prevention), who may be able to take some precautions as a result of this knowledge. For example, it may remind people with asthma to carry an inhaler, or even to change their travel plans.

'Childproof' caps are a health-protection measure aimed at primary prevention of drug poisoning.

Advice to people with high blood pressure about limiting their salt intake is an example of health education at the secondary level of prevention, because it is aimed at reducing the risk in people who are already showing a disease symptom.

2   It is undoubtedly true that such a population screening programme would be costly to conduct; it would have to cover all adult men and women in the UK, and would need to be repeated at intervals to detect people whose blood cholesterol levels have risen since the previous test. Drug treatment for those detected with 'too high' a level of cholesterol would also be hugely expensive; according to one estimate, meeting the National Service Framework target for reducing cholesterol levels in high-risk individuals would cost £1.5 billion per year. The question of effectiveness is harder to answer: a population screening programme would certainly detect and successfully treat a proportion of high-risk individuals who would not otherwise have been identified, so you would expect death rates from CHD to fall as a result of this intervention. However, it will also detect and treat a much larger number who would *not* have progressed to develop CHD if left untreated. The dilemmas raised by such a programme concern the ethics of attempting to compel everyone to be tested, the creation of anxiety in people labelled as 'high risk' by the test but who would not have developed CHD, the prescription of treatment to these people, which itself carries a health risk (as is the case with cholesterol-lowering drugs), and the possible diversion of health funding to this programme at the expense of others that would have delivered greater health gains for a larger number.

3   The first problem is that the classical risk factors *interact*; for example, people who are physically inactive and obese are also likely to have elevated blood pressure and raised levels of blood cholesterol. This makes it difficult to disentangle the relative contribution of each risk factor at a population level, or to determine the most effective prevention strategies for reducing the risks in a given individual. The second problem is in deciding where to draw the line between 'normal' and 'high risk' values for each risk factor; if the line is drawn too low, then prevention strategies will be aimed at a lot of people who will not benefit, whereas drawing the line too high will leave untreated a proportion of high-risk individuals. The third problem relates to the reliability and validity of the research evidence on relative risks and on interventions; studies may have been inadequately controlled, or too small, or have become rapidly out of date in such a fast-moving field, or they may have been biased in the selection of subjects, for example excluding older patients from CHD screening tests or treatment trials.

4   There is a wealth of evidence that the socio-economic and psychological aspects of people's lives have a major impact on their CHD rates. The social class gradient in CHD risk cannot be explained simply in terms of higher exposure to the classical risk factors among men and women in manual occupations compared with those in non-manual jobs; for example, you can see from Figure 8.3 that the gap between them has persisted or even increased over time, despite the falling death rates in all classes. The Whitehall II study found elevated rates of CHD in people who had low self-esteem and low control over their work, even when all the classical risk factors had been excluded. Other aspects that have to be taken into account are issues of access to services and information, which are likely to be less available to people on low incomes, and the effects of stress as a consequence of social exclusion (a subject that we discuss in more detail in Chapter 9). CHD prevention programmes that sought to address complex social factors such as these would have to intervene in employment, social security and income policies, as well as in the organisation and delivery of health and social services.

Chapter 9

1   An absolute definition of poverty is being used here, in which people on lower incomes are described as 'substantially better off' than in the past. Implicit in the statement is the assumption that they can therefore no longer be considered 'poor'. Absolute approaches to poverty can be criticised on the grounds that even if the lower bands of income rise over time, this may not be reflected in rising purchasing power, so people's standard of living does not improve sufficiently to lift them above the 'relative poverty line' of what is considered 'decent' in their own society. It also makes no mention of whether the proportion of the population whose households are living on lower incomes is rising, so there may be a greater number of people affected. Finally, it ignores the effects on society as a whole of the gap in income between the richest and the poorest, which may be increasing even if the lowest incomes are rising. Large inequalities in wealth distribution add to the sense of social exclusion of people at the bottom of the income range.

2   The causes of infant mortality are far more complex than the assertion made in this statement, which could be interpreted as blaming individual women for causing their baby's death through feckless behaviour. An inadequate diet and persistence in smoking during pregnancy are contributory factors in a proportion of infant deaths, but regional variations in IMR (both within and between countries[1]) demonstrate that the strongest predictor is poverty. In households on low income, women are at greatest risk of subsisting on an inadequate diet, partly because they generally have less command over the money (e.g. part-time workers on the lowest incomes are overwhelmingly female), and partly because women tend to go without things themselves in order to maximise what is available for their children. Such households are not generally able to afford the recommended diet during pregnancy, which is based on high quality protein, dairy products, fresh fruit and vegetables. Smoking is a social activity, a response to stress, and an addiction that is harder to overcome in conditions in which few other forms of support are accessible.

[1] International comparisons of infant mortality in high, middle and low-income countries (using the Gross Domestic Product or GDP as a measure of national wealth) are discussed in *World Health and Disease* (Open University Press, 3rd edn 2001), Chapters 2, 3 and 7.

3   In both the market approach to tackling poverty in the 1980s and early 1990s, and in the social inclusion strategies introduced since 1997, there is an emphasis on wealth creation and a rejection of greater income equality as a social goal. Both approaches make the assumption that increasing the level of benefits paid to people who are unemployed or on low incomes reinforces the 'dependency culture'. Both assume that the creation of wealth is an incentive to businesses and entrepreneurs, which will be translated into greater job opportunities and rising wages for society as a whole. Where they differ is that the market approach is based on an *absolute* definition of poverty, which assumes that wealth generation would 'trickle down' to improve the living standards of the poorest. State intervention in the 'market' era was primarily focused on weaning people off welfare by reducing benefits and increasing means-testing, thereby increasing the incentive to seek work. By contrast, social inclusion strategies accept the definition of *relative* poverty leading to disadvantage in education, skills, health, etc., which the state has a duty to redress via initiatives to increase participation in community life. Action since 1997 has focused on enhancing people's employability through education grants, training schemes and local health-improvement programmes, and redirection of the benefit system towards this aim (e.g. welfare-to-work, help with child-care costs, working families tax credit).

4   Wealth has many obvious health advantages, for example in terms of the standard of housing and diet that can be afforded; the ability to access better (or at least faster) health and social services, education, transport and leisure pursuits; the quality of the working environment and 'fringe' benefits for people in highly paid jobs; and the relative freedom from worry about money that causes persistent anxiety among people on low incomes. All health surveys that measure the association with income report that the better-off groups in any society are those with the best health and the longest life expectancies. However, the Wilkinson hypothesis claims that the health of *everyone* is reduced in societies with a large degree of income inequality, i.e. a large gap between the incomes of the richest and poorest. Evidence from societies in which income distribution has become more equitable over time has shown that even the 'richest' sector – in common with everyone else in the society – experiences improvements in health.

Acknowledgements

Grateful acknowledgement is made to the following sources for permission to reproduce material in this book:

Figures

Figures 3.1, 4.1, 4.3, 6.2 and 7.1: Crown copyright material is reproduced under Class Licence Number C01W0000065 with the permission of the Controller of HMSO and the Queen's Printer for Scotland; *Figure 3.2:* Warwickshire Health Authority; *Figure 4.2:* Warner, L. and Wexler, S. (1998) *Eight Hours a Day and Taken for Granted,* The Princess Royal Trust for Carers; *Figure 7.2:* University of Nottingham, Division of Academic Radiology; *Figures 7.3 and 7.4: The Second Annual Report,* The UK Renal Registry, December 1999; *Figure 7.5: Health Care UK 1996/97: The King's Fund annual review of health policy,* Kings Fund Publishing; *Figure 7.6:* Lenaghan, J. (ed.) (1998) *Rethinking IT and Health,* Institute for Public Policy Research; *Figure 8.2:* Reprinted with permission from Elsevier Science, *The Lancet,* Vol 353, May 1999, Tunstall-Pedoe, H. *et al* 'Contribution of trends in survival and coronary-event rates to changes in coronary heart disease mortality: 10 year results from 37 WHO MONICA Project populations'; *Figure 8.4:* McPherson, K., Britton, A. and Causer, L. (2001) 'Monitoring the progress of the 2010 target for coronary heart disease mortality: Estimated consequences on CHD incidence and mortality from changing prevalence of risk factors' in Peterson, S., Rayner, M., and Press, V. (2000) *Coronary Heart Disease Statistics,* British Heart Foundation; *Figure 8.5:* Ebrahim, S., Davey Smith, G., McCabe, C. *et al* (1998) 'Cholesterol and coronary heart disease: screening and treatment' *Quality In Health Care,* **7**: 232-239, BMJ Publishing Group; *Figure 8.6:* Peterson, S., Rayner, M., and Press, V. (2000) *Coronary Heart Disease Statistics,* British Heart Foundation Health Promotion Research Group, University of Oxford; *Figure 8.7:* Hemingway, H. *et al* (2001) 'Underuse of coronary revascularization procedures in patients considered appropriate candidates for revascularization', *New England Journal of Medicine,* **344,** pp. 645-654, copyright © 2001 Massachusetts Medical Society. All rights reserved; *Figure 9.1:* Pantazis, C. and Gordon, D. (eds.) (2000) *Tackling inequalities: Where are we now and what can be done?* The Policy Press; *Figure 9.2:* Wilkinson, R. (1996) *Unhealthy Societies: The afflictions of inequality,* Routledge.

Tables

Table 2.1: Williams, A. (1997) The economics of coronary artery bypass grafting, in Culyer, A. J. and Maynard, A. K. (eds) *Being Reasonable about the Economics of Health,* Edward Elgar Publishing; *Tables 4.1, 5.1, 5.2, 5.3, 5.4, 7.1, 9.2 and 9.4:* Crown copyright material is reproduced under Class Licence Number C01W0000065 with the permission of the Controller of HMSO and the Queen's Printer for Scotland; *Table 6.1:* Centre for Evidence-Based Medicine; *Tables 7.4 and 7.5:* Harrison, A. and Prentice, S. (1996) *Acute Futures,* Kings Fund Publishing; *Table 8.1: Preventive Medicine: A Report of a Working Party of the Royal College of Physicians* (1991), Royal College of Physicians; *Table 8.2:* Prevention, How much harm? How much benefit? 3. Physical, psychological and social harm, reprinted from, by permission of the publisher, *CMAJ* 15 July 1996; 155 (2) (table page 172) pp. 169-176, © Canadian Medical Association www.cma.ca; *Table 9.3:* Lewis, J. and Piachaud, D. (1992) Women and poverty in the twentieth century, in Glendinning, C. and Millar, J. (eds.) *Women and Poverty in Britain in the 1990s,* Harvester Wheatsheaf, reprinted by permission of Pearson Education Limited; *Table 9.5:* Maddison, A. (1989) *The World Economy in the Twentieth Century,* OECD.

Un-numbered photographs/illustrations

Frontispiece, pp. 98, 103, 163 (left), 173, 195 and 211: John Harris/Report Digital; *Page 13:* Michael Abrahams/Network; *pp. 15, 27, 33, 44, 53, 54, 58, 59, 68, 73, 87 (right), 96, 97, 114 and 201:* Mike Levers/Open University; *pp. 35 and 171:* Science Photo Library; *pp. 43 and 106:* United National Photographers (UNP); *pp. 66, 101, 123 and 184:* John Callan/

Shout Picture Library; *pp. 77 and 79:* Lionel Grech; *pp. 81 and 163 (right):* Jess Hurd/Report Digital; *p. 86:* Royal College of Nursing Archives; *p. 87 (left):* Deborah Ratnavel; *p. 122:* Duncan Phillips/Report Digital; *p. 128:* Anthea Sieveking/Collections Picture Agency; *p. 171:* Science Photo Library; *p. 172:* Eye of Science/Science Photo Library; *p. 186:* St Bartholomew's Hospital/Science Photo Library; *p. 191:* Mike Dodd; *p. 197:* Gideon Mendel/Network; *p. 204:* Joy Wilson; *p. 210:* Russell Boyce/Popperfoto.

Every effort has been made to trace all copyright owners, but if any have been inadvertently overlooked, the publishers will be pleased to make the necessary arrangements at the first opportunity.

Index

Entries and page numbers in **orange type** refer to key words which are printed in **bold** in the text. Indexed information on pages indicated by *italics* is carried mainly or wholly in a figure or a table.